CLASSIC PACING

For a better life with ME

Ingebjørg Midsem Dahl

CLASSIC PACING

For a better life with ME

by

Ingebjørg Midsem Dahl

English Edition: Copyright 2018 Ingebjørg Midsem Dahl

ISBN: 978-1-9996418-0-1

This book is produced by Lyngsmyr AS in conjunction with **WRITERSWORLD**, and is produced entirely in the UK. It is available to order from most bookshops in the United Kingdom, and is also globally available via UK based Internet book retailers.

Copy edited by Ian Large

Cover design: Vivian Llarena and Jag Lall

Photo credit author portrait: Hilde Midsem

This edition translated from Norwegian by Ingebjørg Midsem Dahl and Anna Louise Midsem

WRITERSWORLD
2 Bear Close Flats, Bear Close, Woodstock
Oxfordshire, OX20 1JX, England
☎ 01993 812500
☎ +44 1993 812500

www.writersworld.co.uk

The text pages of this book are produced via an independent certification process that ensures the trees from which the paper is produced come from well-managed sources that exclude the risk of using illegally logged timber while leaving options to use post-consumer recycled paper as well.

DEDICATION

To my friends with ME, even those I have not met yet.

TABLE OF CONTENTS

FOREWORD

Ms Dahl has produced a very well written and thorough account of strategies that come under the umbrella title of 'Pacing'. Her approach is very practical and aimed at the whole range of patients, from Mild to Severe. I especially liked her early use of Dr Darrel Ho-Yen's analogy of ME patients having a limited energy budget and how, if they spend it at the same rate as normal people, they will rapidly go bankrupt. I also liked her concept of 'Planned Overexertion', which covers how to cope with something that one has to do that is outside one's energy reserves. She stresses the need for a flexible as opposed to a rigid routine. One of her examples involves a patient who wishes she had adopted a Pacing strategy sooner in the acute early stage of her illness, and feels naturally that this might have spared her some of the length of duration and severity of her illness. I also liked her analogy of running out of energy being like having a flat battery, and how rest is the only way in which energy levels can be restored.

My personal motto for patients who are doing too much has always been "Take two steps backwards in order to be able to take one step forwards", and readers will see that this is entirely in tune with much of the contents of this book.

Ms Dahl rightly stresses that Pacing is not a cure, but more a coping strategy within the limits of one's illness. Failing to adopt a Pacing strategy, especially adopting a rigidly increasing regime of Graded Exercise (GET), is of course almost universally harmful. In the UK patient surveys by the ME Association show that by and large patients favour Pacing regimes strongly over GET.

Ms Dahl's book comes at a propitious time. In the USA, the National Institute of Health has withdrawn all recommendations for Graded Exercise and CBT, and in the UK the National Institute of Clinical Excellence (NICE) is about to review (and quite possibly withdraw) its previous endorsement of GET and CBT. This leaves Pacing as the natural management strategy of choice.

Overall I am sure that this book will prove very helpful for many ME sufferers. Although possibly too detailed for some, it contains something for everyone, and is pragmatic and not over-prescriptive.

Dr Nigel Speight, Paediatrician
Durham, United Kingdom, 2018

FOREWORD FROM NORWEGIAN EDITION

Evidence based practice (EBP) is about using knowledge from research, from one's own experience as a professional, and from the experience of the client. The client's experience represents one of three pillars in EBP. In modern medicine emphasizing the perspective of the client is an important approach, and this is particularly true in medical rehabilitation. This book is an important addition to this pillar because it presents of one of the most important topics for people with CFS/ME, pacing of activities. This book is needed. It is written as a self-help book from one client to another, but it is also important to professionals who want a better understanding of the difficulties clients with CFS/ME face in their daily life.

The author wishes to contribute to increased knowledge of coping skills among other people who have a CFS/ME diagnosis. The information is based on the author's own experience of many years with this illness. She has also collected the experiences of other clients in Norway and internationally. She looks at their experiences in the light of her own, and of some of the available literature.

From the perspective of the clients, the book invites the reader (client) to choose an active approach to their own life situation. The book is conducive to optimism and to believing that it helps to do something yourself. As professionals we have learned, in contact with clients, that they draw benefits from learning about the illness, and about how others have learned to live with it. In the areas where coping courses have been held, experiences have been similar. Experience with coping courses, where they have been able to hold them, tell the same story. At the same time the book presents an approach that the clients themselves recommend – pacing and energy conservation.

Pacing is an approach that suits many, but perhaps not all, as the author herself mentions. Other clients might have objections and other ways of understanding the book's contents.

The book is a self-help book from client to client, but professionals who encounter people with CFS/ME will also find it useful. The book contains many concrete pieces of advice and techniques/strategies that can be used both by the client, and in cooperation with a professional. It can also be read by both parties so as to contribute to a common understanding of the situation.

There is much to interest professionals too. It gives many ideas and experiences that professionals can consider in order to understand what it means to live with this kind of illness. This can contribute to a greater understanding of how one can be of help.

At the same time a professional will disagree with some of the terminology used and some of the interpretations and the understanding of the contents of the book. It must therefore be read in the client perspective that it represents. Then it can be regarded as an important contribution to the development of what will be the future health care for the group of clients with CFS/ME.

BERGEN, 06.02.2014

Bjørg Rene
Specialist in Occupational Therapy

Inghild Follestad
Social Worker

INTRODUCTION

HOW TO USE THIS BOOK

1 Every chapter starts with a summary to make the book more accessible to those with reading difficulties. These summaries can be used either as a quick reminder or to choose the chapters most useful to you.

2 The essentials are in Chapter 1 to help you get started with pacing without having to read the entire book. It does not matter if it takes a long time before you read the other chapters.

3 Read the book in small portions so reading it doesn't make you more ill. The chapters are subdivided into sections to make the book easier to read. Put marks in the margins of the book to remember how far you have read. The best approach is to take your time, both when reading and when trying out the advice.

4 The book is divided into three parts. Part One is about basic pacing, Part Two is about advanced pacing and Part Three has chapters on different themes. You do not need to think about Parts Two and Three before you need them.

5 Every chapter in the book can be read separately like reading an article.

If you have severe ME, you can jump straight from Chapter 1 to Chapter 18, 'Severe ME'. Similarly, you can read the chapter 'Learning, School and Studies' if you are in school or at university.

6 There are tasks at the end of every chapter, which make getting started with pacing techniques easier.

7 You do not have to try everything, and especially not all at once. You get the best results by trying things out, choosing methods freely and putting together a set of management techniques that are suited to your personality, your situation and how ill you are.

8 If your needs change later, or if the first techniques you tried are not enough, you can try out some of the things you did not use first time around.

9 The advice in this book is meant for people with strictly defined neurological ME, but parts of the book can be relevant to other illnesses, including other fatiguing illnesses. Consult a professional if you are in doubt about what could be suitable for you.

WHY TRY SOMETHING THAT IS NOT A CURE?

Pacing is about managing the illness, not about treating or curing it. Some, but not all, experience significant improvement. So what is the point of trying it? Is it not better to wait for a cure?

Numerous doctors have tried to find a cure for ME for over 20 years. Even though some drugs show interesting results, there is still no definitive treatment or cure. A lot of research remains to be conducted before any drugs will be approved for large scale use on ME patients. Therefore, we need something to keep us going while we wait. Pacing and other techniques for managing the disease give us a better quality of life and are available now.

Those who have recovered from ME often say that the things they learned while ill have been useful to them in their healthy lives. Time spent learning pacing is not wasted even if you recover completely. There is nothing to lose and a lot to gain. Bianca Veness, an Australian ME patient states in an article on pacing:

"Using pacing techniques in a flexible way gives me a sense of freedom, as I feel I am listening to and heeding the needs of my body and living with the rhythms of the day, not forcing myself into an unmanageable routine. By staying within my energy envelope, I am liberated from feeling awful, and I can truly enjoy life once again."

ABOUT ME

Myalgic Encephalomyelitis (ME) is classified as a chronic neurological disorder. The World Health Organization included ME in their International Classification of Diseases in 1969 under the code G93.3. The most characteristic thing about the illness is that the symptoms get worse or are triggered by activity, both physical and mental. In severe cases only a very small amount of activity provokes strong symptoms. ME also results in an unusually long recovery time after exertion. Dr. Melvin Ramsay, a pioneer in the field, described this as the "main anchor of the diagnosis". ME causes a number of symptoms from all bodily systems, including neurological, cognitive and muscular symptoms.

ME has been researched for many years by medical professionals, and there have been many abnormal findings. However, most of these findings do not show up in standard tests, which leads to many ME patients being told that their results are normal and there is nothing wrong with them. The findings include: inflammatory processes, disturbances in the immune system, low levels of antioxidants, high levels of free radicals, high levels of nitric oxide and peroxynitrite, leaky ion channels in the cell membranes and defects in the body's stress response. This list goes on.

The disease mechanisms in ME are so complicated that, despite many findings, the scientists have yet to see a complete picture. Because of this, at the time of publishing this book, there is still no diagnostic test. Instead, ME is diagnosed based on different sets of clinical criteria. Comparative research has shown that these different criteria define different patient groups. This complicates research. In the past, the most commonly used were the Fukuda criteria, but they are being substituted by the International Consensus Criteria by Bruce Carruthers and colleagues, because they are stricter and produce a less varied patient group.

ME can affect anyone, both children and adults, women and men. Severity ranges from those who can lead almost normal lives to those who are bedridden, unable to move their own body. Most will be somewhere in between these extremes. In some, the disease enters a latent stage, while in others it is permanently disabling. Many experience improvement, and even people with very severe ME may recover completely. Worksheet 2, 'Activity Scale for Simple Activity Diary' gives you an idea of the range of severity of the disease.

For more information on the disease, read Erica F. Verrio's book, *Chronic Fatigue Syndrome – A Treatment Guide, 2nd edition*. I would also like to recommend *Myalgic Encephalomyelitis – Adults & Paediatric: International Consensus Primer for Medical Practitioners* by Bruce Carruthers et al.

CONTRIBUTIONS

While writing this book I have been in contact with more than 20 ME patients from Great Britain and Norway about their experience with pacing. These experiences are in addition to the hundreds of patient histories I have read in ME publications from several countries over the last 20 years. I wish to thank everyone who has contributed in the making of this book.

SPECIAL THANKS TO THE FOLLOWING:

My mother Anna Louise Midsem for translating this book when it became obvious that it would take too long before I could do it myself, my friend Zoë Williams for proofreading and editorial comments, my medical student cousin Eivind Fosse, for translating the introduction, and my personal assistants, without whom the original Norwegian manuscript would never have moved from my Dictaphone to paper.

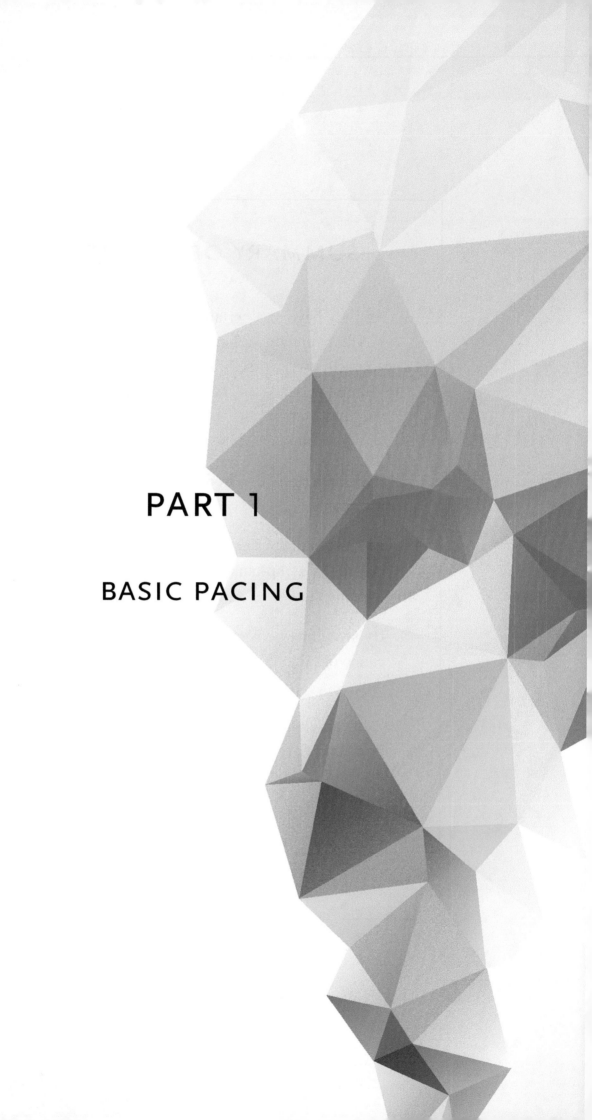

PART 1

BASIC PACING

SUMMARY OF CHAPTER 1

1. Activity beyond a certain limit leads to an increase in ME symptoms. The longer you continue to push yourself, the worse the symptoms will get. The symptoms serve as warning signs, showing that you have done too much. You can experiment gently to find out where the limit is.

2. Rest recharges the body's batteries and reduces symptoms.

3. Avoid symptom flare-ups by stopping all activities before the symptoms become worse, or at the first warning sign.

4. By switching between rest and short activities, you can avoid draining your energy reserves during the day.

5. You can get more out of your energy by switching between physical, social and mental activities, and also between activities that use different parts of your body.

6. Make sure to include some pleasant activities in your day and not just chores and necessities.

CHAPTER 1:

LIVING ON A TIGHT BUDGET

ME — LIVING ON A TIGHT BUDGET

In the early eighties the Scottish doctor Darrel Ho-Yen compared energy to money, and said that healthy people get a hundred dollars a day, while people with ME only get ten, which they have to spread out throughout the day. Recent research has shown that people with ME have several disturbances in energy production in the cells. Therefore, people with ME have less 'energy money' to spend than healthy people. It is necessary to learn how to avoid using more 'money' than you have in order to maximize the chances of improvement. Exceeding the available amount of energy leads to further deterioration of the cells' energy production. How can you avoid doing too much?

UNDERSTANDING ENERGY

One of the most important things is learning to understand energy. In people with ME overactivity leads to symptom increase, while resting leads to symptom reduction. People with ME can begin to feel worse and worse when they take part in physical or mental activities, until they feel so ill that they are forced to stop. Anna from Great Britain gives a good description of it in this quote:

> "I feel really ill, but push myself to crawl out of bed, wash and dress, comb my hair and put on some make-up, since this means a lot to me. Once I am up anyway I feel more motivated and ready to tackle the world. It's this feeling where I think that I ought to push myself more, but soon I start getting warning signs: headache, nausea, dizziness, exhaustion. While I push myself to stay active, I realise that I wasn't that well to begin with, and towards the end of the day I need a lot of help from Mum to undress, wash and get into bed."
> (From *Cheers* magazine, no. 40)

WARNING SIGNS

Note that Anna describes her symptoms as warning signs. That is exactly what they are. The very first, mild symptoms are warnings that show you that you must stop right away because you are about to overdo it. The stronger symptoms that come later are signs that you have already done too much. In Scandinavia people used to say that people who were out of money had pocket pain. People with ME get real pain and other symptoms when the energy account is empty. In the same way that it is a good idea to keep an eye on how much you have left in your bank account, it is important to keep an eye on how much money you have in your energy account.

The most obvious way of doing this is to examine how you feel while you are doing things. As soon as you notice that your symptoms are getting worse, you should stop and rest. The problem is that it is very easy to get so absorbed in what you are doing that you forget to check how you feel. By the time the symptoms are so strong that they interfere with what you are doing, you have already done too much. One possibility is to use the so-called fifty per cent solution that William Collinge describes in his book, *Recovering from ME.* That is about doing half of what you think you can manage. If you think you can walk one kilometre, then you are supposed to only walk half a kilometre. That way you avoid doing too much.

When you use symptoms to decide how long you should do a given activity, it is important to consider all your symptoms, not just exhaustion. Usually, a number of other symptoms turn up before you start to feel exhaustion in your whole body. Some of these can be very mild, like a slight feeling of something protesting in your body.

Therefore, in order to be able to stop in time, it can be simpler to do some concrete experiments that can help you find out where your limits are.

CONSCIOUS EXPERIMENTS

One example of a conscious experiment is to decide to try an activity for fifteen minutes, and set an alarm to tell you when to stop. Afterwards you can evaluate your symptom level. If you feel the same as you did before starting the activity, fifteen minutes is fine. If your symptoms are worse, you try to set a shorter activity time next time. It is a good idea to write down your experiments so that you don't have to try to remember everything. You can copy Worksheet 1 (at the back of the book).

When experimenting, use your previous experience of how much activity you can tolerate as a starting point. If you are exhausted after a two-hour visit from a friend, you should experiment using shorter visits to find the time limit that leaves you still feeling comfortable. If you are bedridden and become worn out after ten minutes, you must experiment with very short activities, preferably of less than five minutes' duration. Perhaps you can read a cartoon, send an SMS, or listen to a song. You will be surprised that you can continue some activities far longer than others, but this is normal. You might be able to read for twenty minutes, but only listen to music for five minutes, or vice versa. You might find that you have to split some activities into very small spells. Maybe you can manage to wash the toilet or the basin or the shower, but not the whole bathroom. Or perhaps you can manage two bites of bread, but not the whole piece. It is not necessary to give up activities just because you cannot go on for as long as other people. Often splitting things up into smaller spells is enough.

REST

When you notice the first warning signs, you should rest. For a healthy person things like watching TV, listening to music or reading, are forms of resting. For people with ME that have less energy to use, those sorts of things must be counted as activities. When you have ME, rest has to be total rest. Rest is not just lack of activity but, in Ho-Yen's money jargon, also the absence of 'spending money'. Rest gives renewed energy in the same way that a mobile phone needs recharging. The best thing is to rest lying down. Many people are too ill to rest sitting up. If you can sit without symptoms increasing, then you can rest sitting for some or all of your rest periods. Choose a comfortable chair that gives good support so that your body can relax totally, and you may find it more comfortable to put your legs up too.

Some people feel that they get the best rest when sleeping, while others find that if they sleep too much during the day, they cannot sleep well at night. A third group feel that they only fall asleep during the day if they are really exhausted and that they don't need to sleep during the day if they get enough rest when awake. No solution suits everyone, so you must find the combination that suits you best.

Not everyone needs much rest during the day. Those who have a mild ME may only need some five minute rests during the day. Those with a 'moderate' degree of ME usually need several long rests and often some short ones in between, too. People who are bedridden need to rest all day, breaking up the rest periods with some short activities. It is important to rest for so long that you feel nice and warm, and actually feel a little better. It is also important that you manage to rest mentally, because thinking takes energy. It is just as important that you have some fixed rest periods, which you stick to no matter how well you are feeling. These give you 'interest on your energy account' and, in time, it may mean that there is 'more money in your purse' if you are lucky.

RELAXATION

The most efficient form of rest is deep relaxation. The point about deep relaxation is that you rest both your body and your mind, instead of your thoughts continuing to grind around in your head. There are many different techniques that you can use. Sometimes one has to try several before finding the one that suits you best. At the back of this book you will find some suggestions as to CDs you can use. I have written more about relaxation in Chapters 3 and 18.

SWITCHING

Switching is important. Resting is not fun. Having to rest for a long time to get over a very long activity period can be very undermining. It is important to have many short activity periods with rest in between, instead of few and long activity periods. It is also a good idea to switch between different types of activities. Doing the same kind of activity all day will easily lead to overworking certain body parts, while others are not used enough. Here is an example of how you can switch between rest and activity, and between different types of activities:

Listening to music 10 minutes – rest 20 minutes

Walk in the garden 3 minutes – rest 20 minutes

Making a birthday card 10 minutes – rest 20 minutes

Reading 5 minutes – rest 20 minutes

In this example the activities are short, and therefore the rest periods are short. The activities use different body parts; in the first activity the ears, in the next the legs, then the arms and finally, the eyes. Some people will need much shorter activity spells and much longer rest periods. Others can manage longer activity spells before they need rest. Even if you can keep going for a much longer time, it is a good idea to split up the activity periods in several shorter spells. For example, you could try doing three different activities of twenty minutes duration each instead of doing the same type of activity for a full hour. You often get less exhausted using this method.

ENJOYING YOURSELF

Enjoying yourself is an important aspect of pacing. It is necessary, since this illness leads to enormous restrictions, that some activity periods are used for things you really like and which make you happy. Some people might say that it is not possible to enjoy yourself doing something for such a short time, like just ten minutes, but it is. It is definitely possible to enjoy yourself, even if just for ten minutes. What is no fun is having to stop. Then it is important to remind yourself that you are stopping in time in order to avoid feeling worse. You are stopping so that you can enjoy yourself again later that day. That way, stopping in time becomes a positive instrument to use, not just a nuisance. Many hobbies and interests can be adjusted so that they can be done by people with different levels of functioning, even from a bed or sofa. Even activities that take place outside the house can often be adjusted so that they need less energy than usual. It is worthwhile looking at new aspects of yourself, or to renew old hobbies that you haven't enjoyed for a long time. Life does not have to be over just because you cannot run a marathon.

OTHER FACTORS THAT AFFECT YOUR ILLNESS

Pacing is not the only positive factor that can affect the health of people with ME, nor is overdoing activity the only thing that can have a negative effect. Overstimulating the senses, stress, infections, food intolerance, hormone changes and weather changes are other factors that can have a negative effect. Coping and treating these factors can help improve your health. It is not unusual for people to discover that using different coping techniques at the same time has a stronger effect than just one technique. However, be smart to just introduce one technique at a time, so you don't get overwhelmed. Part of the reason there are so many other factors that affect the illness lies with the disease process itself. ME affects all organ systems, and creates a complex network of biochemical disturbances. The stubbornness and severity of these vary greatly. This is why competent use of pacing and other management techniques only eases the burden a little for some people, whereas others find that they cause significant improvement in their health.

WHO CAN HELP WITH PACING?

If you find it particularly difficult to learn pacing on your own, it is possible to get help, but availability and quality vary greatly between areas. Part of the reason for this is that national guidelines for the treatment of ME differ. If pacing is not the favoured management strategy in your country it may be difficult to get professional help.

Most healthcare professionals have been trained to help motivate people to try coping techniques, and this may be helpful if you find that lack of motivation to learn pacing is a problem. Occupational therapists and physiotherapists learn basic energy conservation skills in their training. However, many healthcare professionals specialize in completely different areas of their field, and they may lack the experience, interest or knowledge to help you. One of the most common pitfalls seems to be that the professional may get impatient and will push the patient to take on too much activity too soon, which will bring on a relapse. Other patients have received valuable help from professionals who have worked *with* them. One example of this is described in Heidi's patient experience, between Chapters 6 and 7.

Local ME groups usually know whether help is available where you live. Both local and national ME groups may have advisory services and information material, which may be of some help. It can be beneficial to team up with others with ME to learn pacing. You can motivate each other and learn from each other's experiences, cutting some corners in the learning process. There is an online self-help course for people with ME, in which pacing features heavily. The course is available in both English and Spanish and costs very little. You can read more about it on www.cfidsselfhelp.org.

OTHERS CANNOT PACE FOR YOU

Please bear in mind that pacing is essentially a self-management method. The signs and symptoms that are visible to others tend to be signs of overexertion. The early warning signs are usually not noticeable to others. This means we are the ones who have to learn to recognize them and act upon them. Others cannot pace for us. What others may be able to help with is to keep track of our experiments when we have bad cognitive symptoms. They may also be able to help us think of good practical solutions and motivate us to keep pacing even when it is challenging.

THE ADVANTAGES OF PACING

Since ME limits you so much, it can seem like a double punishment to have to limit yourself. That makes it important to focus on the advantages of pacing. First of all, pacing usually makes you feel more comfortable because you stop before you feel really ill. Also, in the long run, pacing provides the conditions your body needs for the best chance of a general improvement. The course of the illness varies depending on many other factors such as infections. However, when you stay within your limits, you may well find they slowly expand. Thirdly, and this is perhaps the most important thing, pacing gives you more control over the illness and, with that, more control over your own life. When you stop in time and rest, you are steering the ME, instead of it steering you. Without pacing it is easy to feel like a passive victim on an endless roller coaster. One doesn't know how one is going to feel tomorrow and therefore planning becomes nearly impossible. With pacing the illness becomes more stable and it is possible to plan which small activities one can enjoy tomorrow. Best of all, you are giving your body what it needs, and increasing your chances of feeling better.

TASKS

1 SENTENCES ON LEVELS OF ACTIVITY

One of the simplest methods of improving your understanding of your own activity level is to formulate sentences about what you can do or cannot do. The sentences can take the form of: *"I feel very ill if…"* or *"I feel ok when…"* For example: *"I feel very ill after having had a visitor for four hours."*, or *"I don't feel worse at all after a telephone call lasting five minutes."* Write down sentences about as many activities as possible. Along the way you might find yourself getting shocked at how little you can do. That is quite common. Try to think of the sentences as an instrument for efficient pacing. That way they become instruments to make you better, instead of making you feel depressed.

2 A FORM FOR THE EXPERIMENTS

It is practical to have a form to use where you can write down your experiments. 'Worksheet 1' has been made especially for this. Take a look at the sentences you made in Task 1 and transfer what you already know to the form. Using the examples I used in Task 1, you can fill in 'four hours' under the activity 'social life' and the column 'severe symptom increase'. Under 'telephone calls' you can put 'five minutes' in the column for 'no symptoms'. When you have put in what you already know, you can begin to experiment and fill in the gaps in the form. You experiment by deciding ahead of time how long you will spend on an activity. Then you evaluate how you feel during and after the activity and put the results in the form. Using the previous example, if you get severe symptoms after having a visitor for four hours, then try one hour and see if you then avoid symptom increase. The goal is to find out how much you can do without an increase in symptoms. You must only experiment on the areas covered by the first two or three columns. Experimenting with things that give you severe symptom increase or relapse will just make you more ill. Only fill in the columns for severe symptom increase and relapse if you end up doing too much by mistake.

3 SET PACING GOALS

When you have a fair idea of what you can do without symptom increase, try to stick to activity periods of a length that have been shown to not worsen your symptoms. Instead of setting goals for what or how much you should do, try to set concrete goals about staying within your limits. This is especially important in activities where you have a tendency to keep going for too long. It is easier to stop in time if you know that that means you are reaching today's goal. This way you get the advantages that accompany goal-setting without risking overdoing things or having a relapse. Pacing goals should be concrete, like having a certain number of rests, and you should choose a number of goals that you have a chance of reaching. If you set goals about always stopping in time, you are sure to end up feeling a failure. It will not always be possible to stop in time, but you can have good effects from pacing anyway.

It is also possible to set goals for bad days, such as, "If I'm not well enough to phone a friend, I'll text instead." This can help you feel like you are on track, even on bad days.

KARINA, 30 YEARS OLD

"I am one of those who has had ME for 5 years. I became acutely ill after mononucleosis when I was 25. I went from working fulltime as a nurse and 20,000 steps a day, to 22 hours in bed. I was too ill to read, and knew nothing about ME or pacing. I have become gradually better during the past 5 years. I still get flu-like symptoms from too much activity, but I feel almost totally well if I just rest and stay on the sofa.

My best pacing tips are:

— Switching between different activities. Don't do the same thing for too long at a time. If you can read for 5 minutes without getting worse, you read for 2.5 minutes before you do something else.

— Rest (in bed with no stimuli) for 20 minutes, for example every other hour, also on good days. Use an alarm clock to warn you when it is time to rest. I feel ill if the rest lasts for too long. I now have mild ME, and can manage without rest during the day. But I can have a higher activity level if I rest several times during the day.

— I have to keep my pulse under 60. I started walking to the children's day centre with my youngest son when I was moderately ill. Then I walked 100–200 metres before I took a rest. My experience is that I can walk further, if I walk very slowly and take small breaks along the way.

— Visualising was very important for me during the worst periods. I went through the walk to the WC in my head before I did it, and that way it went a little better to get to the toilet. I also visualised nice hikes in nature that I had enjoyed earlier, and that made my body more relaxed.

— I tackled sounds I knew better. For example, I could listen to known quiet songs on the iPod, to isolate myself from the crying and screaming of my 1-year-old baby.

–   Rest before doing tiring activities, and take lots of rest afterwards, too.

– Use your energy on pleasant activities. Let other people do the housework, so that you can play a game with the children or read a book.

I wish I had been given simple information on ME and pacing during the acute phase, because I pushed myself the first half a year, because I didn't understand the illness and was very poorly cognitively. With the right treatment during the acute phase, that is pacing, I think I could have reduced the risk of developing a chronic illness."

SUMMARY OF CHAPTER 2

1. Choosing energy-efficient ways of doing things means you can get more out of your available energy.

2. Keywords for saving energy:
   - comfortable position
   - leisurely pace
   - technique, rather than strength
   - one thing at a time
   - split tasks into small pieces
   - use energy-saving appliances and aids
   - simplify tasks
   - remove background noise and anything that interferes with concentration

3. Energy-saving appliances from ordinary shops include a thick pen, mobile phone with touch screen, electric toothbrush, wheeled shopper or a backpack for shopping. More tips can be found at the back of the book in Chapter 23: 'Tips for Energy Conservation'.

4. Some of the most common aids that people with ME find helpful are wheelchairs, office chairs with brakes for use in the kitchen, and shower seats. In some countries these can be borrowed through an occupational therapist, mobility centre or charity.

5. If you have assistance needs over time, apply to the state for assistance if possible.

CHAPTER 2:

ENERGY CONSERVATION

INTRODUCTION

Energy conservation is an important technique for people with ME because it allows us to make the most of the limited amount of energy we have. The principle is similar to power saving – if you use less electricity, it costs less and you have money left over, which you can spend on other things. Or to put it another way, if you use less energy in your daily routines, then you have more energy left to do things you enjoy.

Energy saving is simply about finding less strenuous ways of doing things. For example, it is less strenuous to sit than to stand. If you set yourself up so that you can sit in those situations where people usually stand, you save energy, which can then be used for other things. Energy conservation cannot replace the other principles of pacing: splitting activities into small enough sessions so that symptoms do not get worse, and taking rest breaks between sessions, so as to charge the batteries. Nevertheless, energy efficiency does enable us to get more out of the energy we have.

THE MAIN PRINCIPLES OF ENERGY CONSERVATION

Use these points as a guide when creating your own energy efficiency measures:

1. Choose the least strenuous working position for each activity.

2. Simplify tasks.

3. Reduce background noise and anything that interferes with your concentration – do one thing at a time.

4. Reduce your speed.

5. Refine your techniques rather than using brute strength.

6. Use energy saving devices/aids.

ENERGY SAVING TIPS

There are a large number of tips in Chapter 23. Here we will look at a few of the most common tips.

CHAIR OR PERCHING STOOL IN THE KITCHEN

One can save a lot of energy by having a high chair or stool in the kitchen that you can sit on while cooking or washing up. There are office chairs with wheels and brakes, so you can decide when to roll and when to stand still. A standing support chair is an office chair which provides proper height and angle when working at a kitchen worktop. A perching stool gives the same height and angle, but does not have wheels. What you prefer is a matter of taste. You may be able to borrow both types through an occupational therapist. It is possible to ask to try both before deciding.

SHOWER SEAT IN THE BATHROOM

It is possible to save energy in the bathroom by sitting on a shower seat. In the bath, one can use a so-called bath board, which is a seat that goes across the bathtub. A stool or chair can also be used in front of the sink, for example, when brushing your teeth.

TABLE FOR BED OR CHAIR

There are several types of tables you can have on your lap when sitting in bed, in an armchair or on a sofa. One type is a beanbag tray. These are easy to handle and can be used anywhere, but the tray tilts when you move your legs. Another type of table stands on the floor and goes over the chair or bed. These tables are sturdy enough to be used if you want to paint, eat soup or do other things that require a strong surface. The tray can be purchased in stores like Ikea, while you may be able to borrow a bed/chair table through an occupational therapist.

WHEELCHAIR AND SCOOTER

ME often limits walking distances. If you have to say no to things because you cannot walk far enough, you might benefit from a wheelchair or mobility scooter in those situations. There are many different types of wheelchairs and scooters. Some are small and easy to transport in a car, others are larger and suitable in places with difficult terrain. An occupational therapist may be able to help assess what you need, and organise for you to try out different types. Since self-propelling a wheelchair is a major strain on the arms, electric wheelchairs, power chairs and scooters give the greatest freedom of movement. There are some small models that can be transported in a normal car.

BOOK HOLDERS AND AUDIO BOOKS

If you struggle to read because it is difficult to hold the book or magazine, you can try out different types of book holder, including some that can be used lying down. For concentration problems, you can try audio books. They can be expensive, but can be borrowed for free from the library, and some countries have postal libraries of audio books for disabled and chronically ill people. To join you may need a note from a doctor, nurse, or occupational therapist. Audio books can be played on MP3 players and computers. Some audio libraries have streaming apps for smartphones. DAISY format is designed to make it easier to navigate audio books, which is useful for studying.

FINDING THE RIGHT EQUIPMENT

Occupational therapists know about the different types of aids available, and how to obtain them, and they may be able to arrange for you to borrow some equipment for free. In some countries these are available from the National Health Service. In other countries, you'll need to see them privately, but insurance companies may cover the cost. Examples include a tray to wash hair in bed, or tin or jar openers that are easy to use. There may be short-term loans, which are useful for relapses, or long-term loans. The processing time for long-term loans varies. Therefore, one should apply as early as possible, and children should apply for new aids before they have outgrown the old one. In many cases, there are several aids to choose from, so you can get something that fits your own body shape, the size of your home or the terrain where you live. It is worth looking through a catalogue or website with different aids to get an idea of what is available.

In those countries that do not have a national health service, it may be possible to borrow aids from various charities. There may also be grants you can apply for, to enable you to buy equipment. In most countries it may be possible to rent equipment short term, but for long-term use it will be cheaper to buy equipment second hand.

ASSISTANCE

Delegating tasks to others can save a lot of energy.

If you have paid assistants it leaves your family, friends and acquaintances free to facilitate you with more enjoyable or important activities without having to worry about the more mundane tasks.

Assistance can enable you to rest adequately and so have the energy to do something nice, instead of all your energy going on essential jobs. However, the use of assistants needs to be carefully planned so that the benefits do not disappear in the effort required to use the assistance.

If friends and family ask if there is anything they can help with, you can create a list of odd jobs and hang it on the fridge. Then they can look at the list to see if there is anything they can help with. Examples of such tasks may be putting out the rubbish or recycling, washing up, mowing the lawn or washing windows. You can split your list into tasks that take minutes or tasks that require more time.

Some places have volunteers who can assist with things like getting to a doctor's appointment, making a large batch of dinner to freeze, or a large shop. Volunteers cannot be used to cover substantial assistance needs, but you can use them if you just need assistance once in a while, or to supplement more regular assistance.

SUBSTANTIAL ASSISTANCE NEEDS

If you need assistance for a long time, you should apply to get assistance from the state if possible. This avoids wearing out your friends and family. There are a variety of community services for people who are sick and disabled, but they are different in different countries. All services have advantages and disadvantages and it is important to study carefully the various services before applying. It is also important to think about your needs before the assessment, in order to present them in a way that the assessor can understand. For example, although you may be able to shower yourself, to do so may leave you so exhausted that you cannot have an outing, or see a friend. The assessor may not be used to this kind of disabling illness, so you will need to explain this. Explain that in order to be able to do a certain thing you need assistance with another, such as food preparation or showering.

Forms of assistance that are provided in some areas include: personal assistance (to help with all aspects of daily living), home nursing (for more medical care needs), respite care (for short-term breaks), home help (for household chores) and meals.

Whatever type of assistance you have, it pays to make weekly plans and/or daily schedules, because this saves a lot of effort. Arranging the day's schedule so that you alternate between tasks you need to be involved with, and things the assistant can do alone gives natural rest breaks. When you pay for your assistance yourself you can get exactly what you want and can write your work lists accordingly. With state assistance this may not always be the case. Some local authorities have very strict rules as to what home nurses and home carers are allowed to do, and you may find that they are only allowed to do exactly the tasks you've been granted. Some of your nurses/carers may still be flexible, but others may be very rigid. To avoid being drained by unnecessary conflicts you need to base your work lists on what they're allowed to do. Personal assistance tends to be more flexible than home care even when it's covered by the state.

The list should be written as keywords, not text, otherwise there is a danger that assistants feel that they have insufficient time to read it. Moreover, the list should be written in the first person ('I', not 'he/she') even if a family member writes it. This is done to highlight the fact that people with ME are people with their own opinions, not objects to be cared for.

****

The energy saving tips mentioned in this chapter are just a small sample of those that exist. A larger selection can be found in Chapter 23: 'Tips for Energy Conservation' at the back of the book. You can also find more suggestions for energy conservation measures at www.metips.co.uk. With a little creativity, you can find your own energy conservation measures. Write them down and share them with others.

TASKS

1 Consider how the specific energy efficiency suggestions in this chapter apply to you.

2 Consider your daily activities and how these can be done in a less strenuous way.

3 When you feel ready to try new energy conservation measures, see Chapter 23. Read just a small section, make a list of a few measures that suit you, and try them one at a time. Later you may want to read more of the chapter and make a new list.

SUMMARY OF CHAPTER 3

1. Cognitive (intellectual) problems like memory problems or concentration problems are symptoms of ME: the symptoms get worse if you use your head and/or your body too much.

2. Cognitive problems can get better if you rest your mind enough and switch between different activities. That way you don't wear out your brain all the time.

3. Relaxation techniques can make it easier to rest your brain.

4. It is easier to concentrate if you cut down background noise and remove other things that disturb you.

5. One kind of cognitive problem is mental overstimulation, which is all about your brain becoming so exhausted that you cannot calm down your thoughts.

6. If cognitive problems make it difficult to pace your activities, there are solutions worth trying, for example making a routine or using a timer to remind you to stop.

CHAPTER 3: COGNITIVE ACTIVITIES

CHAPTER 3:

COGNITIVE ACTIVITIES

INTRODUCTION

Problems with thinking, concentration and memory are also called cognitive problems. These are symptoms of ME. Cognitive problems affect pacing in two different ways. First of all, cognitive problems get worse with effort. This can be reduced by avoiding overdoing things. Secondly, cognitive problems can make pacing difficult. We will look at both of these aspects in this chapter. Cognitive problems also affect learning. You can read more about that in Chapter 17, which has to do with learning, school and studies. Chapter 17 is also relevant to people who are not at school or taking courses. In Chapter 23 in the section about Reading, Writing and Communication, there are some good tips that ease cognitive problems in these areas.

PACING OF MENTAL ACTIVITIES

Let us first look at how you can pace mental activities. An important part of pacing is choosing peaceful activities that don't exhaust you too much. These could be activities like listening to music, watching TV or reading. What these activities have in common is that they are mental and need concentration. If you do these most of the day or in most of your activity periods, you will quickly find yourself in a situation where your physical symptoms are improved, but your mental functioning is worse. The solution is to pace your mental activities, not just the physical ones. This means stopping all activities before symptom worsening occurs. You also have to make sure you get mental rest and vary your activities as much as possible.

GETTING MENTAL REST

The vital step is to make sure you get several rest breaks during the day, where you also rest your brain. You can use relaxation techniques or sleep. It is also possible to rest the usual way, while making sure that you avoid thinking too much. You can empty your mind, let your thoughts pass by without hanging on to them, and feel peace settle around you. After a while you might choose to imagine that you are lying in a beautiful spot in nature, or imagine that one part of your body at a time feels heavy. Many people feel that relaxation sessions are a good way of reaching mental rest. Relaxation can be learned in several ways.

You can listen to CDs with instructions, or read instructions in a book. You can learn relaxation directly from a professional or at a course. In the task part of this chapter there is a relaxation session you can try. At the back of the book there is a list of relaxation resources. It can take a little time to learn relaxation, particularly if you have strong symptoms or are very tense. If you have a lot of problems learning relaxation, you should ask a professional for help.

SPLIT UP MENTAL ACTIVITIES

Besides mental rest, it is also very important to split up mental activities into small chunks so that one avoids getting symptoms from them. Healthy people experience quiet activities like watching TV as rest. To people with ME these are activities, because they cause exhaustion. For that reason these, too, must be limited in order to improve symptoms. This is no fun, and it is easy to be tempted to go for too long. Remember, it is more fun to watch TV for half an hour and avoid feeling worse afterwards than going on for three hours and ending up with a terrible headache.

The most important thing is to split up everything into small pieces and vary activities. Normally you do not have to give up the activities entirely. If you find it difficult to split up the activities, or stop in the middle of things, choose activities that are self-limiting to some degree. For example, you can read books with jokes or quotes, poems or short stories instead of novels. You can listen to one song instead of the whole album, and choose audio books that are easy to split into small portions, such as sketches and short stories. As for TV, you can experiment with short films, series with short episodes and the like.

Most TV programmes can be watched in two sittings, but it is often difficult to split them into smaller pieces. If you try to see a two-hour film in 15-minute sessions, you will usually lose track of the story. For this reason, a better solution is to split a half-hour programme into two if you can only watch for 15 minutes.

Humour programmes with sketches can be cut into even smaller bits because you can stop the video/DVD between two sketches. Nikki, a British woman with ME, says:

> *"I have given some things up. I can't watch subtitled movies all the way through, and it's just not as much fun when you have to break the suspense and spread a film out over days. But there aren't that many things you can't break into little bits and still not get a lot out of them. Some things actually improve for having breaks in between because you have time to think about the best way to continue before you go back to them."*

MAKE SURE YOU VARY THE ACTIVITIES

Variation is also important. In ME, mental activities do not only lead to mental symptoms and physical activities to physical symptoms. Physical overactivity can lead to mental symptoms and the other way around. You can avoid this by doing appropriate amounts of physical and mental activities without overdoing either of them. If you can manage to do an activity for a while, you will most probably be less exhausted by doing several short things after each other instead of one thing for a longer time. For example, you can watch TV for 20 minutes, do a craft activity for 20 minutes and read for 20 minutes. After a rest you can do the round once again. You can also try some low-energy activities other than the purely mental ones. Many craft activities are good for this. You use a very different form of concentration when you lay a puzzle, build Lego or make birthday cards than you do when watching TV and the like. If you don't know which craft type you might like, you could borrow craft books at the library or look at catalogues and magazines.

DO ONE THING AT A TIME

Healthy people have no problem holding a conversation while the TV is on in the background. People with ME find this difficult or totally impossible. Even if you manage to do it, you will get exhausted twice as fast as if you watch TV first and chat afterwards. Reducing distractions and doing just one thing at a time can greatly reduce cognitive problems. Turn off the TV, radio and PC except when they are actually in use. Close doors, and use ear plugs. Flashing lights and things that move are also distracting. If necessary, remove flowers that smell, reduce draughts, and make sure to keep the room at a comfortable temperature with pleasant lighting.

If you must do something that takes extra concentration, it may be necessary to sit at a table that is completely empty except for the things you are actually using for that explicit task. People who become distracted by text and pictures on the page they are reading can make a reading prosthesis, as recommended by the neuropsychologist Linda Miller Iger. This is a piece of thin cardboard where one cuts out a long, thin opening. The opening must be as high as one and a half line, and as broad as the text in the book. When you put the reading prosthesis on top of the text, you can only see one line at a time and therefore cannot get distracted. If you have a lively family, it might be difficult to be with all of them at once in the room. Get them to join you in another room for short periods, or just some of them at a time. Try to find out which activities you can do with them, like lying on the floor and drawing.

MENTAL OVERSTIMULATION

Most people think of cognitive problems as slow thought processes. It is not as well known that you can experience thoughts that rush past. Thoughts grind around in the head and can't be stopped. This is called mental overstimulation. Mental overstimulation can make it difficult to pace activities because one feels 'geared up' and can't manage to rest. It can help to try to stop all activities before you become overstimulated and to use relaxation techniques when you rest. Mental overstimulation is described in more detail in Chapter 12.

HOW COGNITIVE PROBLEMS CAN MAKE PACING DIFFICULT

Concentration and memory problems can make pacing difficult in several ways. You can forget that you had planned to rest, or forget to check whether it is time to stop. Concentrating on a conversation can take so much out of you that you can't manage to find an appropriate ending to the conversation. You can also forget to write in your activity diary, if you have one, or make too many appointments during a week because you forgot that you already had one. These difficulties may perhaps sound like bad excuses for not pacing your activities well enough, but they are very real. However, there are several tricks that can make things simpler.

STRATEGIES YOU CAN USE WHEN COGNITIVE PROBLEMS GET IN THE WAY OF PACING

STOPPING IN TIME

- Decide ahead of time how long you want to stay at an activity, such as listening to three songs. It is easier to remember how many songs you have heard, than to try to judge how long you can manage to keep listening.

- Timers are a good idea, that is if one can remember to turn them on.

- Try to choose activities that are so short that you can finish them in one go. Make it a habit to rest when you have had the one go.

- Have a flexible daily routine. This saves the effort of planning.

- If you have problems remembering the routine, get someone to write it down on a piece of paper in a clear way that is easy to read. Put the paper where you can easily see it.

MAKING APPOINTMENTS

- Use an appointment book in order to avoid overbooking.

- Make it a habit to check the book every time someone wants to make an appointment with you.

- Most mobile phones have a calendar function that you could use and it can remind you of your appointments.

ENDING CONVERSATIONS, VISITS AND PHONE CALLS

- Tell people ahead of time how long you can manage to have a visit or talk on the phone. Repeat this when people arrive.

- Use the timer too and tell people that you feel less ill when you avoid overexertion. That increases your chances that your guests might actually leave (or end the call) when the alarm goes off.

- The responsibility of keeping a social activity within your limits should not be left exclusively to others. The social situation becomes much simpler when people are prepared for the visit to be short.

REMEMBERING THE ACTIVITY DIARY

- Take the diary with you everywhere and put it in a very visible place if you choose to write an activity diary for a period.

- When using a detailed activity diary, write down the time you start an activity, and then the time you finish it. That way you don't have to remember how long you have been at it.

- In the beginning it is normal to forget the diary. Use a reminder on your cell phone until you have established the habit.

*****

If none of the above mentioned techniques help, give your brain all the rest it needs. As one begins to get better, the cognitive symptoms usually improve so that you can begin to think clearly again.

TASKS

1 Start using several daily rests that give you total mental rest.

2 Make sure you stop mental activities in time, so that you do not get a flare up of symptoms.

3 Learn at least one relaxation technique in order to improve your mental rest. A list of relaxation resources can be found at the back of the book. Here is a simple relaxation session of the autogenic training type that you could try: Lie on your back with eyes closed in a quiet room. Breathe deeply and peacefully with your stomach. When the body begins to feel quiet and heavy, think of one part of your body at a time. Think: "My right arm is heavy, my right arm is heavy." When it actually begins to feel heavy, you change to the left arm and think that it is beginning to feel heavy. Do this with all your body parts. As the body quietens, you can imagine that you are resting in a pleasant place, or something else that you connect with peace and being comfortable, like stroking a cat, or drinking a cup of cocoa.

4 Make sure you have good variation between physical and mental activities.

5 Consider how your cognitive symptoms make it difficult for you to pace your activities. Find strategies to lessen the problems.

SUMMARY OF CHAPTER 4

1. An activity diary is a tool you can choose to use to improve your insight into what you can manage to do and what you cannot, in order to prevent bad days.

2. A simple activity diary is used to evaluate the activity level from day to day. This type of activity diary is good for long-term follow up.

3. In a detailed activity diary you can see all the activities during the day. This type works best for shorter periods of time.

4. With a simple diary you can draw a graph that shows the connection between your activity level and your symptom level. You judge the activity level on one scale and the symptom level on another. See Worksheet 2.

5. A detailed diary is interpreted by asking questions. For example:

   - Does the activity give worsening of symptoms?

   - Are the rest breaks used to get over overdoing it, or to keep your energy up during the day? Are there clear patterns? For example, that you get worse and worse throughout the day?

6. A simple diary can make it easier to stick to activity pacing long-term, because you can see from the graph that your plan actually works.

CHAPTER 4:

THE ACTIVITY DIARY — AN IMPORTANT TOOL

INTRODUCTION

"You have a bad day again and you can't imagine why. Was it the trip to the shops yesterday that did it? You stopped early on purpose to avoid overdoing it. Or was it Aunt Gerda's visit the day before yesterday? Or something totally different? Who knows? You turn over in bed and try to get some more sleep."

It sounds so simple, doesn't it? Overdoing leads to relapse. In ME the reaction to doing too much can come as much as three days later. That makes it difficult to keep account of what really led to the bad day. In the first chapter, energy was compared to money. An economist would say that the first step towards control over your economy is to find out what you are actually using your money on. This means you should keep an account of it. It is possible to keep an energy account too, in the shape of an activity diary. Using an activity diary makes it easier to find out which activities and combinations of activities work out well and which don't. The knowledge you get from the diary can be used to prevent the bad days. This chapter is all about how you make and interpret two different types of activity diaries, a simple one and a detailed one. In Chapter 6 you can read about how you can use the activity diary to make a routine that works both on good and on bad days.

IS IT NECESSARY TO KEEP AN ACTIVITY DIARY?

An activity diary is an optional tool. Pacing is not about keeping a diary, but is about using symptoms both as a measurement of how much you can do, and how much healing rest you need. Not everyone has the physical or mental capacity to keep a diary, not even if they dictate it instead of writing. Luckily, it is perfectly possible to pace without using a diary. It is very intrusive to have other people keep your diary for you – it can be an invasion of privacy. Family or healthcare personnel should not keep a diary for people with ME, unless the person with ME has explicitly asked them to. If you want to keep a diary but can't manage to do it yourself, it can still work well for someone else to do it for you. In that case it is necessary that you trust the person and feel that you have control over the project yourself.

SIMPLE DIARY

In a simple diary you judge the level of activity on one scale and the symptom level on another. The diary makes it possible to see how the two are connected. If you overdo it, your symptoms get worse and the level of activity gets lower until you are better. If, on the other hand, you stay within your limits, the symptoms may well decrease gradually over time. You judge the level of activity on a scale from 0 to 100, where 0 is no activity and 100 is normal activity. The scale is on Worksheet 2. The symptom level is judged on a scale from 0 to 10, where 0 is no symptoms and 10 is very strong symptoms. You can see an example in Figure 1. You can keep your diary on Worksheet 3. A simple diary is necessary for making a flexible routine of the type described in Chapter 6. Since a simple diary is easy to keep, it lends itself nicely to long-term use.

FIGURE 1 — NEHA'S SIMPLE DIARY

	ACTIVITY LEVEL	SYMPTOM LEVEL	NOTES
MONDAY	70	4	Good day
TUESDAY	70	6	Wired, hard to relax
WEDNESDAY	40	7	Pretty tired
THURSDAY	30	9	Completely exhausted
FRIDAY	40	7	Little better today

DETAILED DIARY

In a detailed diary you note the time and how long all activities and rests last during the day. You also judge your symptom level on a scale from 1 to 10 before and after every activity. A detailed diary can be used to find out how long you can continue to do your different activities, and whether the activities are spread out during the day in a suitable way. You may discover that there are some activities you cannot do on the same day, or that you collapse in the afternoon because you do too much in the morning. Figure 2 shows an example of a portion of a detailed diary. In this example, John's grandmother comes to visit and stays for three hours. Afterwards, John feels much worse and even after an hour's rest he still doesn't feel as well as he did before his grandmother came. It is obvious that it would be better to have a shorter visit next time. You can keep a detailed diary on Worksheet 3. Since it is demanding to have to write down all activities and times during a day, this system works best when used for shorter periods of time. If you want to be able to see how your activities develop over time, you can choose to keep the detailed diary every now and then, for example once a month or four times a year.

FIGURE 2 – EXCERPT FROM JOHN'S DETAILED DIARY

SYMPTOM LEVEL BEFORE ACTIVITY (0-10)	TYPE OF ACTIVITY	TIME	SYMPTOM LEVEL AFTER ACTIVITY (0-10)
5	Lunch	14:00-14:15	5
5	Rest	14:15-14:30	4
4	Visit from Grandma	14:30-17:30	8
8	Rest	17:30-18:30	6

ELECTRONIC DIARY

It is possible to keep an electronic diary in the calendar function of mobile phones. On a smart phone you can download different types of health diaries. One of these, 'ME Diary', has been made specifically for people with ME: ME Diary makes it easy to register symptoms and activities, but you can only register blocks of 30 minutes' duration. The system is therefore more suitable for people who are well enough to continue with activities for that long.

OTHER DIARIES

Some people feel it is worthwhile to keep a diary of other factors that can affect the health of people with ME. Such factors could be stress, sleep, food, menstruation, or weather conditions. If you think you might benefit from this type of diary, you should avoid keeping a diary where you register all the things at once. Take one thing at a time.

A BIT ABOUT INTERPRETING A SIMPLE DIARY

The point of keeping a diary is to gain insight into which activities you can tolerate. If you don't feel you are gaining that insight, the effort of keeping the diary is wasted. That is why interpreting it is important.

The easiest way of getting a general view of the simple diary is to draw a graph. You can draw a graph on Worksheet 5, 'Graph Sheet for Simple Activity Diary'. The activity level and the symptom level are drawn on the same graph so that you can see how they affect one another. In Figure 3 you can see a graph of Neha's activity diary, which was shown in Figure 1.

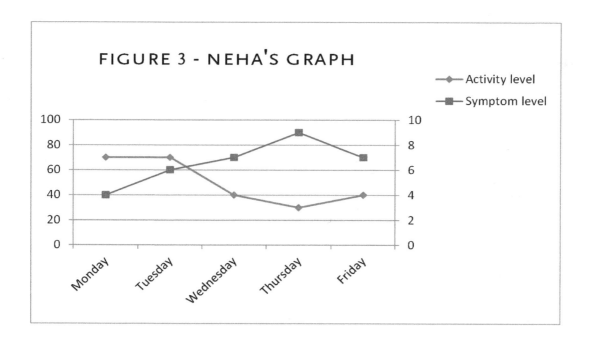

On the good days, Monday and Tuesday, Neha does a lot. Tuesday she begins to feel worse, and by Wednesday the symptoms are so bad that she has to do much less. On Thursday she can hardly bear to do anything. Friday, after having had some rest, she begins to feel better again. If Neha had done less on Monday and Tuesday, for example activity level 50, she would probably have avoided the bad days towards the end of the week.

Pacing your activities cannot stop all the bad days, but if you avoid overdoing it, you are likely to experience fewer bad days, and the bad days will be less awful.

A BIT ABOUT INTERPRETING A DETAILED DIARY

When you interpret a detailed diary you don't use a graph, you use questions. It is also possible to colour your diary to get a better overview. You can have one colour for rest breaks, one for main activities and one for less demanding activities. You can read more about main activities and less demanding activities in the next chapter. In the book *Mindfulness for Health* by Vidyamala Burch and Danny Penman, they suggest a third method. Here you fill in Worksheet 6. This sheet has three columns. One is for worsening of symptoms, one for unchanged symptoms and one for improvement of symptoms. You put each activity in the correct column in the diary. A list like that gives a good overview of what is too much, and what is a suitable length. Figure 4 shows an example on the analysis sheet that has been filled in from John's activity diary in Figure 2.

FIGURE 4 — JOHN'S ANALYSIS SHEET

+ WORSENING OF SYMPTOMS	0 NO CHANGE IN SYMPTOMS	— IMPROVEMENT OF SYMPTOMS
Visit from grandmother 3 hours	Lunch 15 minutes	Rest 15 minutes Rest 1 hour

In Chapter 16 you will find a list of questions you can use when you interpret a detailed diary.

The questions can be used, whether or not you want to use an analysis sheet. Here you can see the most important:

1. Does the activity lead to an increase in symptoms?

2. Are the rests used to recuperate from overdoing it, or to retain your energy throughout the day?

3. Are there clear patterns, for example getting worse and worse during the day?

Let's have another look at the example about John in Figures 2 and 4. The answer to the first question is that John does not get a worsening of symptoms after lunch, but that he gets strong worsening of symptoms after the visit that lasted for 3 hours. The rest after lunch is used to retain energy, but the long rest after the visit is used to recuperate after overdoing it. Also, the visit creates a peak in the activity level, which is followed by a dip in the shape of a long rest. The conclusion is that a fifteen-minute lunch suits John well, but that a visit of three hours is too long. This example may be so simple to grasp that one perhaps could have done without the diary to draw this conclusion. However, if you are going to study a whole day, then it is much easier to retain an overview when everything is down on the paper in front of you.

USING A DIARY IN THE LONG TERM

When improvement takes a long time, the diary can be an important motivational factor. Figure 5 is an example based on my own activity diary. The dots on this graph do not represent days, they represent a month's average. The graph shows two years of my life. The activity level is kept constant, while the symptoms gradually get better. When improvement is as slow as this, it is easy to forget how you felt some months ago, and you can end up thinking that you are not getting better. A diary can enable you to see that you are managing to stick with pacing, and that it works. That way you avoid losing hope. Of course, improvement does not always come as slowly as it did in my case, even in people who are as ill as I was.

Be aware that the diary does not necessarily show all changes. One example of this could be that you began to rest sitting up, but that you forgot to write it in the diary. On looking back you could be awfully disappointed in not seeing any change, when the truth is that you can sit far more than you used to. The danger of not registering changes is greatest in the simple diary. You can reduce this risk by being careful to write all the small or large changes on the notes line in the diary.

You can also choose to keep a detailed diary sometimes. Then you have to make sure to register all activity in the diary. Otherwise you won't see the changes here either. If you follow this advice, everything should fall into place to make the diary become a tool for motivation instead of a disappointment. That way the diary can become a useful tool, both in the short, and the long term.

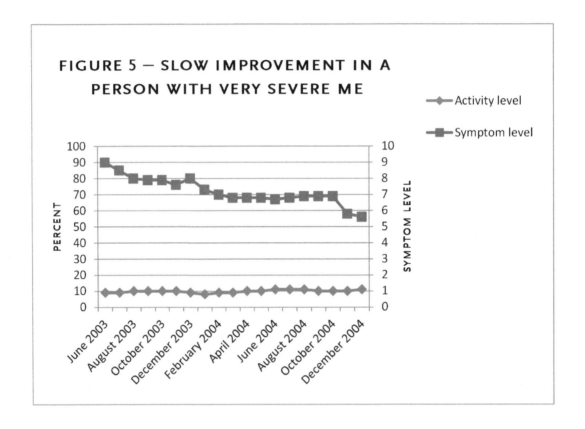

****

Using a simple activity diary for several years is not only an important tool in coping, but it also gives solid documentation of the fact that the coping techniques you use, actually work. The most important thing you gain from keeping an activity diary is that you learn to understand the connection between your activity level and symptom level. This improves your chances of organizing your life so that you get as many good days as possible and, hopefully in time, gradual improvement. In other words, you get more control over your life. It takes a bit of an effort to get started on the diary, but once you have, your efforts are rewarded.

TASKS

1 Start keeping an activity diary. Use one of the two enclosed sheets, or make your own.

2 Think about whether you need different aids for keeping your diary. These might be:

- keeping a simple diary instead of a detailed one.
- a Dictaphone, so you can dictate instead of writing.
- a diary you can take with you everywhere so that it is always within sight.
- leaving a note on the table, or using the reminder function on your phone, to remind you to fill in the diary.

3 Interpret the diary with the help of a graph or of questions, depending on whether you have chosen a simple or a detailed diary.

4 Use the information in the diary to find out what you can change in order to prevent bad days and symptom flares during the day. Make the changes a little at a time if necessary.

SUMMARY OF CHAPTER 5

1. What I call 'main activities' are those that are a little more demanding than the ones you spend most of your time doing. What the main activities are depends on the severity of the disease.

2. With less demanding activities you may be able to keep going for longer than with main activities.

3. You can often get more out of your energy by finding a good balance between the main activities, less demanding activities and rest. Typically, this means that one must have only a few main activities, and keep them short.

4. It may be that what you currently think of as your main activities are actually too strenuous. If that is the case, you will need to consider your activity level – do you need to cut back? Some of the activities you've been considering less strenuous may actually be your 'main activities' and need to be upgraded in your mind to give them the importance they require.

5. When you have ME and the limited amount of energy that goes with it, it's important to prioritise where this energy is spent. This can be done by creating four lists: things you must do; things you want to do; tasks that can be delegated to others to do; and those you do not need to do.

6. When one wants or needs to do something that is really too much, and will make you more ill afterwards, there are ways to make it easier. You can take extra rest beforehand, adapt the activity to use as little energy as possible, and rest a lot immediately afterwards. This kind of planned overexertion should be rare, in order not to wear down your level of health.

CHAPTER 5:

MAIN ACTIVITIES AND PRIORITIES

INTRODUCTION

When you have a limited amount of energy, it is important to distribute your activities in a way that enables you to get the most out of the day. In addition, one must prioritise any vital tasks. We will look at both in this chapter.

MAIN ACTIVITIES

Some activities are more strenuous than others. Main activities are those that are a little more demanding, of which you can manage maybe one or two a day. The most demanding activities that one can only do once in a while are discussed in the section entitled 'Planned Overexertion' later in this chapter. What is a major activity depends entirely on how sick you are. For a person with moderate ME, a main activity might be a visit or a shopping trip, or maybe an hour or two of education. If you are severely ill with ME, meals are often a major activity, and so is being washed in bed. A full working day or a picnic with the family can be the main activities for a person with mild ME. These are only examples, and it will be different for different people. Even people at around the same level of illness will find different activities more or less tiring depending on their particular mix of symptoms and abilities.

EXAMPLE 1: NEHA'S MAIN ACTIVITIES

Neha has moderate ME. In the previous chapter we looked at her activity diary. Figure 1 represents the diary with main activities. Notice that Neha's main activities are distributed very unevenly across the week. In the next chapter we will look at how to redistribute the main activities to try and reach a more stable situation.

FIGURE 1 — NEHA'S MAIN ACTIVITIES

MONDAY	TUESDAY	WEDNESDAY	THURSDAY	FRIDAY
Doctor's appointment	Ironed bed linen	Visit by friend	Rested on sofa	Yoga class for people with ME
Laundry	Paid bills			
Walked to the corner shop	Dusted			
Made dinner	Made dinner			

	MONDAY	TUESDAY	WEDNESDAY	THURSDAY	FRIDAY
NOTES	Good day	Wired, hard to relax	Pretty tired	Completely exhausted	Little better today
ACTIVITY LEVEL	70	70	40	30	40
SYMPTOM LEVEL	4	6	7	9	7

EXAMPLE 2: PETER'S MAIN ACTIVITIES

Peter is bedridden. His main activities are short and take place in bed. For people with milder degrees of ME, Peter's activities would be undemanding activities but for Peter they are major because he is very ill. Notice that Peter has divided his activities so that he alternates between physical, mental and social activities.

FIGURE 2 — PETER'S MAIN ACTIVITIES

MONDAY	TUESDAY	WEDNESDAY	THURSDAY	FRIDAY
Body wash in bed 10 min	Internet 10 min	Phone call 5 min	Hair wash in bed 10 min	Audio book 10 min

CHAPTER 5: MAIN ACTIVITIES AND PRIORITIES

EXAMPLE 3: HANNA'S MAIN ACTIVITIES

Hanna has mild ME and is well enough to work 28 hours a week. As with Peter, Hanna only has one main activity a day, but her activities are much more strenuous than either Peter's or Neha's.

FIGURE 3 – HANNA'S MAIN ACTIVITIES

MONDAY	TUESDAY	WEDNESDAY	THURSDAY	FRIDAY	SATURDAY	SUNDAY
Work for 7 hours	Work for 7 hours	Qigong class for people with ME	Work for 7 hours	Work for 7 hours	Shopping with family, max 2 hours	Visiting friends with the family, max 4 hours

UNDEMANDING ACTIVITIES

Undemanding activities are peaceful activities that you are well enough to do for a longer time than the main activities. People with moderate and mild ME are often able to do less demanding activities for large parts of the day. With severe ME however, it is common to find that even these activities are curtailed. Audio books, radio, computer, TV, reading and gentle hobbies are among the activities most often found less tiring. For people who are severely ill, looking at clouds or daydreaming might count as undemanding.

DISTRIBUTION OF ACTIVITIES

One can use the distinction between 'main activities' and 'undemanding activities' to distribute activities throughout the day. If one does too many main activities too close together, people with ME usually find that their energy is used up very quickly, and it will trigger a flare up of symptoms. It is important to rest before the symptoms flare up. However, if you choose to have few main activities in short sessions, with less demanding activities and rest in between, then one can find that the available energy lasts longer. It is the severity of the disease which determines how many activity periods you can have, and for how long, and how much rest you need.

EXAMPLE 4: GEIR'S DISTRIBUTION OF ACTIVITIES

Figure 4 shows Geir's morning. Geir is moderately ill, but at the more severe end. He finds activities like showering, cleaning and gardening tiring. When he has done these activities for half an hour, he must rest for an hour afterwards before he is able to continue. In Figure 5, Geir started to switch between the main activities and undemanding activities. This means that he showers one day and cleans the next, but he is no longer so exhausted by the activities that he must rest for a long period afterwards. Geir's redistributed morning is just an example – there are many possibilities and you must try until you find the one that works best.

FIGURE 4 – GEIR'S MORNING

WHAT	HOW LONG
Showering and cleaning	30 min
Rest	1 hour
Gardening	30 min
Rest	1 hour
Lunch	15 min

FIGURE 5 – GEIR'S REDISTRIBUTED MORNING

WHAT	HOW LONG
Shower	15 min
Internet	15 min
Rest	15 min
TV series	30 min
Rest	15 min
Gardening	15 min
Audio book	15 min
Rest	15 min
Browse a gardening book	30 min
Rest	15 min
Lunch	15 min

WHEN THE MAIN ACTIVITIES ARE TOO STRENUOUS

You may find that the activities that you currently think of as main activities are actually too strenuous, and that you need to redefine some less tiring activities as your main activities. Cassandra Wall discovered this. She writes:

> "I thought I had adjusted my activities to do as much as I could, then rest as long as I needed. But no. I was told I'm always at the limit of what I can do, and it was maintaining my exhaustion. First I cut out many things that had pushed my limits: A 90-minute yoga class, a two-hour drive to visit relatives, talking on the phone for an hour, and sometimes a one-mile walk. I cut down to 15 minutes of TV (The National ME Centre was classing TV as a demanding activity), maximum one hour with friends, or 20 minutes on the phone, and only a five-minute car ride. These were my daily limits. All other activities I did in 10-20 minutes, then rested for 40-50 minutes. What happened was that for the first time in many years I began to feel properly rested."

Being forced to redefine undemanding activities as the main activities is not fun, but as the quote above shows, it can still improve quality of life. No longer pushing yourself to the limit can help you to feel less ill, and in the long term it can also help improvement. Cassandra experienced significant improvement during the next five years after she learned how to avoid overexertion.

PRIORITIZING

When a person has ME, usually their energy is very limited, and they want or need to do more than they really can. It is important to prioritize so that you get done what you need to do, and have some energy to do what you love. To get an overview of one's priorities, the book *Setting the Pace* (by The Shropshire Enablement Team) suggests that it is useful to create four lists: one of tasks that must be done, one of tasks one likes, one of chores others can assist with, and one of tasks you do not need to do. Among tasks that need to be done are eating, toileting and some degree of personal hygiene. If you live alone and lack assistance, various types of chores also fall under this. If these tasks are more than you can manage, even if you use energy conservation measures, or if they leave you with no energy left for the things you love to do, it is definitely worth applying for some form of assistance.

FIGURE 6 — NEHA'S PRIORITIES

THINGS NEHA HAS TO DO	THINGS NEHA WANTS TO DO	THINGS OTHERS CAN DO	THINGS NEHA DOESN'T NEED TO DO
Laundry	Make dinner	Vacuum	Ironing bed sheets
Pay bills	Yoga class	Large shopping trip	
Dust	Have a visitor	Other heavy cleaning	
	Walk to the corner shop		

Figure 6 shows Neha's priority lists, based on her main activities from Figure 1. In reality, it may also be necessary to take undemanding activities into account. Neha is married but has no children. She and her husband have divided the housework so that Neha does the least energetic tasks, which are easy to split into short sessions, while her spouse does the heavier tasks such as vacuuming and shopping. Neha puts her housework tasks on the list of things she has to do, while her husband's tasks are on the list that others can do. Neha loves cooking, and she wants to cook twice a week. Therefore, she puts this on the list of tasks she enjoys. Other people might put this on the list of what they need to do, or a task they can delegate to someone else. Also, having a visitor, doing yoga and shopping at the corner shop are pleasurable activities for Neha. She has decided to consider ironing of linen as unnecessary. In the next chapter we shall see how Neha uses priority lists as a basis for creating a routine.

PLANNED OVEREXERTION

In some situations, you may want (or need) to do something that you know you are not well enough to do without getting an increase in symptoms. This might be because your daughter is getting married, or perhaps a visit from a professional if you have severe ME. If you know in advance that you are going to overexert, you can follow this recipe:

FIGURE 7 – RECIPE FOR PLANNED OVEREXERTION

A	Make sure that you get lots of extra rest for a week or two before the strenuous activity. Any preparations, such as packing and organising a trip, should be done before this rest period.
B	Use energy-saving measures to make overexertion and exposure to sensory stimuli as small as possible (see Chapters 2, 20 and 23). Common solutions include lying down, using a wheelchair, sunglasses or an eye mask, ear plugs and asking for a quiet space at an event.
C	Rest as much as possible immediately afterwards. It is better to try to rectify overexertion and exposure very quickly, rather than feeling ill for several weeks.
D	After the event, gradually increase activity back to your normal routine when you feel well enough. Even if you think you are well enough to go straight back to doing everything you normally do, it pays to make sure you are fully recovered from the exertion first.
E	Wait a while before you plan another overexertion, to reduce the risk of relapse. Planned overexertion is not something to do all the time – ideally, one should not have more than a few planned overexertions during a year.

If the overexertion was not planned, you can still follow points C to E.

Be aware that unusual activities are likely to tire you more quickly, even if you have planned and paced everything carefully. You can read more about this in Chapter 7, 'Improvement and Increasing Activity'. With good and realistic planning it will often be possible to implement planned overexertion without causing long-lasting consequences. However, there are situations where it is best to say no because the effort would be too great. It is not a good idea to implement planned overexertion regularly, as there is a risk of undermining your level of health.

CONCLUSION

An understanding of your main activities, undemanding activities, priorities and how to plan an overexertion are all tools to effective pacing. These tools can make it more possible to spend your energy on the things that are most important to you, without doing too much. As usual there is no solution that fits all – you will need to find the combination that suits your particular situation.

TASKS

1 What are your main activities at the moment? You could write them on the memo lines of Worksheet 3, 'Simple Activity Diary'.

2 Which undemanding activities do you like doing?

3 Consider if the main activities are too strenuous for your current level of health, and whether any of the less demanding activities should be defined as main activities.

4 Prioritize your activities. You can use the 'priority sheet' (Worksheet 7) for this. Try to include as many aspects of life as possible.

5 Next time you know beforehand that you will overexert yourself, try to follow the recipe for planned overexertion. Attempt to organize it so that planned overexertion is something that happens only rarely.

SUMMARY OF CHAPTER 6

1. It can be easier to stay within your limits if you have a flexible routine. In order for a flexible routine to have this effect, it must be planned so that all activities are kept within your limits. How strict a routine you need depends on your situation, personality and how ill you are.

2. A flexible routine can be adjusted as needed, and that is an advantage.

3. A rigid routine can be difficult to combine with the necessities of daily life.

4. Before you make your routine, you should keep a simple activity diary for at least two weeks and decide which activities to give priority. See Chapters 4 and 5. There is a short step-by-step explanation of how to make a routine in the 'Tasks' paragraph.

5. You can ask for help if you find it difficult to make the routine yourself.

6. The strictest routine will not necessarily produce the fastest improvement. It is better to make a routine that you are happy with, so that you can stick to it over a longer period.

CHAPTER 6:

A FLEXIBLE ROUTINE

INTRODUCTION

A flexible daily routine is an optional tool like the activity diary. A flexible routine can be adjusted to suit any life situation, personality and degree of illness. At times a relatively loose routine could be best. During other periods things may work better using a strict routine, where large parts of the day are planned in detail. This applies especially if you are having trouble stabilising your condition. In this chapter we will look at the advantages and disadvantages of a routine, and at how to make a flexible routine. Following a routine does not actually have anything to do with pacing. You are only pacing if the routine helps you to stay within your limits.

ADVANTAGES OF A FLEXIBLE ROUTINE

Having a flexible routine has several advantages. It is easier to make plans if you have a framework. When you plan a realistic amount of activity each day, you can avoid the bad days and prevent exertion-related relapses. Also, it helps to know what you are going to be confronted with. Starting on something and then having to stop in the middle of it, can feel like a defeat. But knowing that you are only going to be busy with the task for, say 15 minutes, it is easier to feel proud of what you have managed to do in the time. You can do a little each day, and manage to get through big projects without relapse. A condition for making a flexible routine work is that it is set up so that when you follow it, you are staying within your limits.

DISADVANTAGES OF A RIGID ROUTINE

A rigid routine means that you have to do the same thing every day at a given time. Routines like these are difficult to combine with normal daily life, because they leave no room for unforeseen events. Also, it can quickly become boring. Some people do experience the need for a strict routine for a period of time. This probably applies mainly to those with very severe ME. Sarah, a young British woman who has had ME for a long time, says:

> *"First I tried to pace my activities strictly, but it didn't work. I couldn't take into consideration my family's and friends' activities, nor could I include the unpredictable things that happen in life. Pacing is meant to help, so if you don't feel relaxed and comfortable with the way you are doing it, you are doing it wrong."*

When you have ME, you don't live in a vacuum. You are a part of the world for better or worse. Therefore, good pacing is not just about realistic planning, but is also about changing plans when unexpected things happen. That way you can avoid overexertion.

PREPARATIONS FOR MAKING A ROUTINE

Before making a routine, you should keep a simple diary with main activities for at least two weeks (see Chapter 4). Afterwards you prioritise which activities you want to use your energy on (see Chapter 5). It is risky trying to make a routine without keeping the diary ahead of time. You may end up making a routine based on the amount of energy you hope you can cope with and not the amount of activity you can actually manage. If you choose to make a routine without having kept a diary, make sure the activity level in the routine is well below the amount of activity you normally do. You can always increase your activity later if it turns out to be too low. You can read more about improvement and increasing your activities in Chapter 7. If you would like to make a routine for a full day, you should read Chapter 15 first.

FIRST STEP: SPREAD THE ACTIVITIES

The first step is spreading the activities in the routine out over different days. It is easier if you write each activity on a piece of paper so that you can move them around and try out different combinations.

Activities should be distributed according to the following principles:

1. Spread the activities evenly. Avoid doing too much some days and nothing other days.

2. Find a good balance between physical, mental and social activities, and also between enjoyable and laborious tasks.

3. When placing activities that are more demanding, you should partly plan extra rest, and partly make sure that the next activity is less demanding.

4. All activities must be kept within the limits you can tolerate. See Step 2.

Below you will find the rest of Neha's example from Chapters 4 and 5. If you would like to see other examples, look at Chapters 5 and 12.

EXAMPLE 1: NEHA'S ROUTINE

When Neha makes her plan she starts by studying her notes on what she did last week (see Figure 1, which is the same as the one in Chapter 5, 'Main Activities and Priorities'). The most obvious thing is that the activities have been spread very unevenly. On the good days, Monday and Tuesday, she has four activities, but this leaves her so exhausted that she can only manage one activity on Wednesday and none on Thursday. On Friday she is a bit better and can manage her yoga class. Neha decides to use the 50 per cent solution, as described in Chapter 1. Since she thinks she can manage four activities on a good day, two will probably be enough, so Neha plans two activities every day. The 50 per cent solution may not suit everyone. Some people may find it works better to take what they can manage on a pretty bad day as a starting point. In Neha's case that would mean one activity per day.

When distributing her activities, Neha takes into account that activities outside the home are more tiring than indoor activities. For this reason, she plans a trip to the doctor, one to the nearest grocery shop, and her yoga class, on three different days. She also tries to arrange the two daily activities on the same day so that they are of two different types. On Wednesday, for example, she chooses to dust, which is a physical activity, and to have a visitor, which is social. The finished routine is shown in Figure 2.

FIGURE 1 — NEHA'S MAIN ACTIVITIES

MONDAY	TUESDAY	WEDNESDAY	THURSDAY	FRIDAY
Doctor's appointment	Ironed bed linen	Visit by friend	Rested on sofa	Yoga class for people with ME
Laundry	Paid bills			
Walked to the corner shop	Dusted			
Made dinner	Made dinner			

	MONDAY	TUESDAY	WEDNESDAY	THURSDAY	FRIDAY
NOTES	Good day	Wired, hard to relax	Pretty tired	Completely exhausted	Little better today
ACTIVITY LEVEL	70	70	40	30	40
SYMPTOM LEVEL	4	6	7	9	7

FIGURE 2 — NEHA'S ROUTINE

MONDAY	TUESDAY	WEDNESDAY	THURSDAY	FRIDAY
Doctor's appointment	Walk to the corner shop	Dust	Pay bills	Yoga class for people with ME
Laundry	Make dinner	Visit by friend	Make dinner	Visit by friend

SECOND STEP: THE LENGTH OF ACTIVITIES

The second step in making a routine is to make sure that the total routine does not exceed your limits. Every activity in the routine must be kept so short that it does not lead to symptom flare-ups. If you have filled in the experiment form that is mentioned in Chapter 1, you can use this as a starting point. It can also be helpful

CHAPTER 6: A FLEXIBLE ROUTINE

to use the analysing form (Worksheet 6 from Chapter 4, 'The Activity Diary – An Important Tool') if you have filled it in.

EXAMPLE 2: NEHA'S TIMING

Neha knows from experience that she can manage a one-hour visit with no problem, so in the routine she writes down that she can only have visitors for an hour. She spreads out activities like folding clothes and dusting in smaller pieces. Every time she has been at it for ten minutes, she lies down on the sofa and listens to an audio book. This way she avoids being worn out. She also uses energy conservation techniques. For instance, she sits on a chair while making dinner, and she chooses simple meals that do not take a long time to make.

The total number of activities during a week must stay within one's limits. If you drop activities towards the end of the week because you are exhausted, it usually means that you have planned too many or too long-lasting activities – unless it is obvious that other factors are the reason for feeling worse. The routine must be planned so that you can <u>comfortably</u> get through all the activities.

THIRD STEP: ADD REST BREAKS

Adding rest breaks to the day's activities is an important tool for avoiding overexertion during the day and week. Neha takes a half-hour rest after every main activity. In addition to this, she rests for ten minutes every hour. A person with mild ME may only need five minutes rest per hour, while someone with severe ME will usually need far more than Neha. Remember that the point of the rest breaks is to preserve your energy throughout the day, and is not about recuperating after having done too much. If and when something unexpected turns up, or you have to do a main activity that is more strenuous than usual, you should take extra rest. Remember too, that you should take the rest breaks on the good days too, even when you feel you could manage without them. This gives you that bit of extra margin that increases your chances of having several good days in a row.

FOURTH STEP: CONSIDER THE LESS DEMANDING ACTIVITIES

Last, but not least, you should make sure that you also pace the less demanding activities that you will be doing in between the main activities. Having main activities that are short enough for you to avoid symptom increases will not be of much help if you are wearing yourself out on little things you do in between them. Thinking that less demanding and varied activities can be kept short and rotated during the day can be helpful.

FIFTH STEP: PLAN POSSIBILITIES FOR VARIATION

The fifth step is to plan for having variation in your routine. Sometimes, exchanging a planned activity with another you would rather do is a good way to avoid getting tired of the plan. The important thing, if you want to try this, is to make sure that the new activity is not more demanding than the original one. This might mean that you have to spend a shorter time on the new activity, or that you have to exchange two less demanding activities for one short, but more strenuous activity, and a rest. On a bad day you can choose to do less demanding activities than those on your plan. If you have problems remembering how long you can do different activities without getting symptoms, you can make a list.

You can also plan how to tackle the more demanding activities that are not done every day, like shopping and visits. These activities shouldn't lead to symptom increases the same day or the following days. This often means that you can only do these activities for a very short time even when using energy conservation techniques. This is no fun. But it is still important to hang on to the thought that there is much to gain from not getting worse from fun activities. Besides, the change may only be temporary. If and when you get better, you can increase your activity level. Let's look at an example of how to plan variation.

EXAMPLE 3: HOW NEHA PLANNED FOR VARIATION

In Neha's routine she has planned a doctor's visit on Monday morning. But Neha does not have an appointment. She would like to have a different activity outside the house during the weeks when she does not have to go to the doctor's. She decides to spend half an hour at a café those weeks. Should Neha have an appointment with the doctor on a different day of the week, she can switch the activities around. If the doctor's appointment is on Tuesday, she can shop on Monday. On the other hand, Neha knows that Wednesday's dusting and doing the laundry are both physical activities, which should not be done on the same day. So if she has her doctor's appointment on Wednesday, she should move yet another activity to maintain a better combination. The yoga class on Friday cannot be moved. If Neha has a doctor's appointment on Friday, she has to drop the yoga class. She decides to avoid doctor's appointments on Fridays if possible.

SIXTH STEP: TRY OUT THE PLAN

Try out the routine for a few days. It often takes several days to get used to a new routine. You might notice right away that the routine is too demanding. Don't be too disappointed if this happens. People with ME tend to overestimate how much they can do. Instead, you should use your new knowledge to set up a new and less demanding routine. Whatever you do, don't hang on to a routine that is too demanding. That will only lead to relapse. Even when your new routine seems very easy, you should wait several weeks before you attempt to increase your activity level. How you can do this is explained in Chapter 7.

IF YOU CANNOT MANAGE TO MAKE THE ROUTINE YOURSELF

Some people find that their concentration is so bad that they need to structure their day in order to avoid overexerting time and again. At the same time their concentration may be so poor that they cannot plan a routine themselves. It is perfectly possible to ask others for help. It can feel very intrusive that others have an opinion about how you should live your life. For that reason it is important that those around you don't try to push you into letting them help you plan your routine. If you would like help, it is important that you yourself decide who the helper should be. The best thing is to choose someone you trust and who will co-operate well with you. A health care professional may not be better at this than someone who knows you well.

****

You don't necessarily get the quickest improvement by choosing the strictest routine. The best result occurs when you find a routine that suits your body, your soul and your situation. Sarah, whom I have referred to earlier in this chapter, says: *"Pacing is very personal. If you don't do what works for you, it is meaningless to try, since you won't be able to keep it up in the long run."* You can try out different degrees of structure until you find the right combination. The goal is not to refrain from all activities, but an everyday life that works well while staying within your limits.

TASKS

1 In preparation for planning a flexible routine, you should keep a simple diary with main activities for a minimum of two weeks and decide which to give priority to. See Chapters 4 and 5.

2 Make the actual routine. Spread the main activities out over the day and week. Avoid doing too much one day and too little another. Make sure to balance physical, mental and social activities, and also work-like and enjoyable tasks.

3 Make sure the routine does not exceed your limits. The main activities must be so short that they do not lead to symptom flare-ups.

4 Plan fixed rest breaks. The rests should be used to maintain your energy during the day, and not to get over overexertions.

5 Less demanding activities between the main activities must not drain your energy. It helps to vary activities.

6 Plan opportunities for variation so that you don't get tired of the routine. Make sure that the variations stay within your limits.

Try out the routine. If it gives symptom increases, the activity level is too high. Adjust as needed. If the routine suits you, read Chapter 7 before you think about increasing the activity level.

HEIDI, 26 YEARS OF AGE

"My experience is that the healthier I get, the more difficult it is to pace. There are so many things you want to do and have to do. It is very important to avoid excesses as much as possible. I have made friends with many people with ME who are roughly as ill as I am, and most feel that the backlash after doing far too much is worth it and live accordingly.

I really believe that in reality the thought of it being worth it becomes dangerous, because the perspective is too short. When you experience that it 'only' takes a day or two of rest after doing too much, it becomes easy to repeat the pattern and that can hinder improvement in the long run. The important, fundamental improvement is difficult to appreciate because it happens so slowly, while the improvement after overexertion comes quite quickly.

I have also thought about this a lot. The memory of a good experience can keep me going emotionally for a long time, and that it is worth it to have some bad days in exchange for a really good day. The psychologist, who helped me with my pacing, made things clear for me with this eye-opener:

He likened pacing in ME to chemotherapy treatment in cancer.

He said that a cancer patient is willing to go through a very difficult treatment and take all the painful consequences of the treatment in the hope and belief that it in the end would make them healthier.

He said that many ME patients are not willing to go through the pain and sorrow of having to go without the pleasurable and spontaneous activities for a period, even though they know by experience that it will make them better in the long run.

I had to practise refraining from important activities and accept feeling sad about it, instead of doing the activities and accepting being made worse by them. He gave me a simple rule during my first appointment (easy to remember, difficult to do):

The activities that you do, you must be able to do every day without getting worse/needing more rest.

I paced myself before I started seeing the psychologist, but back then I had a plan for my week that included 'swim 500 metres' once a week. I had been doing that quite a while and thought that it was working well. When the psychologist asked whether I could do the swimming every day, the answer was no, I had to have a quiet day both before and after the swimming. I stopped doing the activities that I could not have managed every day, including the swimming, and after a few months the brain fog lifted."

SUMMARY OF CHAPTER 7

1. You must have an improvement in symptom level before it is possible to increase your activity level without the risk of a relapse.

2. It is very risky to increase your activity level when you have an infection or are exposed to other stressors.

3. When you are ready to increase your level of activity you must only increase one activity at a time. Increase the activity by a maximum of 10% at a time.

4. Switch between increasing physical, mental and social activities. Concentrating on only one activity is inadvisable.

5. Increasing activity too quickly or too suddenly can result in relapse. Let your symptom level go down a bit between each increase.

6. In the beginning you should wait several weeks between every time you increase the activity level. Later on you can experiment with quicker increases, if your illness has not reacted badly to previous increases.

7. People with ME cannot force themselves to health by increasing activity level, as if they were simply unfit. You cannot force improvement; you need to be careful and listen to your body.

CHAPTER 7:

IMPROVEMENT AND INCREASING ACTIVITY

INTRODUCTION

Once you have used pacing for a while, and the symptom level has begun to go down a bit, you are probably ready for an activity increase. This is a challenging stage in your illness because it is not always easy to tell when it is safe to increase. The general advice in this chapter is true for all levels of functioning, but for those with severe ME it can take a considerably longer time to reach the stage of being able to increase. For them it is very important to show extra vigilance while increasing activity. It is very important to read the chapter on severe ME before trying to increase your activity level, because people with severe ME are living with very little leeway.

In this chapter we will look at how you can increase your activity level in a sensible way, and when it is safe to increase. Let's first look at the warning signs that show us when not to begin increasing.

WARNING SIGNS

Figure 1 lists the warning signs that indicate caution is needed and activity should not be increased. The first three signs on the list are high symptom level, unstable condition and relapse. All three can be signs telling you that you are close to the limit that you can tolerate. You may even have crossed the line. In that case it would be very risky to try to do more. When you are close to your limit, it can help to do less and rest more for a period of time. This gives your body the opportunity to recuperate. If you are uncertain about how to do this, you can read Chapter 1. Infections, allergies and strong emotional stress are additional strains. When you are considering increasing your activity level, you should include an evaluation of any extra stressors. If you are under any additional strains, your body often needs some extra energy to cope with them, and that makes it risky to increase your activities. It is better to wait until your body is back in balance again. If you simultaneously increase your activities and try out new foods to see if you tolerate them, it will be difficult to know whether any reaction has to do with the increase or the food. It is therefore not a good idea to do both at the same time. It is better to try out the new food first. If that goes well, you can increase your activity level a few days later. Later, perhaps after a week or so, you can try a new food again.

FIGURE 1 – YOU SHOULD NOT INCREASE YOUR ACTIVITY LEVEL WHEN:

- You have a high symptom level.
- The illness is not stable.
- You are getting sicker and sicker.
- You have an infection or an allergic reaction.
- You are trying out new foods to see if you can tolerate them.
- You are under strong emotional strain, or exposed to any additional strain.

WHEN IS IT SAFE TO INCREASE YOUR ACTIVITY LEVEL?

You do not have to be free of all symptoms before you begin to increase your activity level, but it is very important that the symptom level is on its way down. Fewer symptoms and a lower intensity of symptoms mean that you are on the move away from your upper tolerance limit. If you start to increase activities before the symptom level has begun to fall, there is a great risk of overexertion, and overexertion can lead to relapse. That is not advisable. It is safe to increase when your condition is stable, the symptom level is on its way down, and you are not subject to extra stressors. You can find a reminder in Figure 2.

FIGURE 2 – IT IS SAFE TO INCREASE ACTIVITIES WHEN THESE THREE REQUIREMENTS ARE FULFILLED:

- Your condition is stable.
- The symptom level is on its way down.
- You are not under additional strain.

HOW OFTEN CAN YOU INCREASE THE ACTIVITY LEVEL?

Improvement in your symptom level is the main factor in deciding how quickly activities can be increased. If your symptoms are improving slowly, the increase in activity must be as slow. The rule is that your symptom level must go down at least one notch between every time you increase your activity level a notch. This way you keep your surplus energy and avoid draining your resources. You should give yourself enough days between increases to be able to tell whether the increase was too much. That way your body will have enough time to get used to the new activity level. A long time could pass before your body is ready to do more. When the improvement comes you might only be able to increase twice a year to begin with. Before you are able to increase as often as once a week, you must be getting better at a noticeable rate. Even when improving quite quickly you should not increase more often than every third day. This is because you will not otherwise be able to check how you are doing between increases.

HOW MUCH SHOULD I INCREASE?

It is important that the increases are so small that they are hardly noticeable. The reason for this is that bigger increases which are tiring drain your resources. This can slow down the improvement process. In Great Britain it is usual to advise increases of around 10%. This means that an activity of, for example, a five-minute duration can be increased by a half a minute. A ten-minute activity can be increased by a minute, and an activity lasting 60 minutes may be increased by six minutes. If the spells are very short they can be counted by seconds instead of minutes. It is a good idea to set an alarm in order to be certain to stop at the right time.

The main advice is to increase only one activity at a time. If your condition is improving very quickly, the best solution may be to make small increases to several activities at the same time. It can be less strenuous for the body to spread out an activity increase thinly over several activities.

Figure 3 lists the best way to increase activity.

FIGURE 3 – HOW TO INCREASE:

- Let the symptom level go down at least one notch before your increase the activity level one notch.
- Increases should be small, approximately 10%.
- Increase only one activity at a time.
- Vary the increases between physical, mental and social activities.
- Put off an increase if you are having problems.

If the increases make you tired it is a sign that you are increasing your activity level too quickly or too abruptly.

WHICH ACTIVITIES SHOULD YOU INCREASE?

You should switch between increasing different types of activities. This could be physical, mental or social activities, or also activities where different body parts are involved. You do this in order to avoid over-using certain body parts or functions. The greater the variation, the better. No matter what you do, some activities will always be more taxing than others. People with severe ME should start by increasing the least tiring activities because this gives the lowest risk of relapse. Those with moderate or mild ME can choose to increase moderately strenuous activities, but should wait a while before attempting to increase the more exhausting activities.

When you increase the more energy-intensive activities you should be especially careful. It is very important not to increase this kind of activity until you feel that it is natural to do some more. Remember that the usual rules for pacing also apply when increasing activity. This means, among other things, that you should stop before you feel worse or get symptoms.

DIFFERENT STRATEGIES FOR INCREASING ACTIVITY

How you increase activity in the beginning depends on what sort of activity level you already have. Persons with mild or moderate ME would usually spread their activities in the course of a day more or less like this: many less demanding activities (sofa activities), a few rest breaks and a few more demanding activities, also called main activities. You can read more about main activities and less demanding activities in Chapter 5. If you are in this group it is important not to reduce the amount of rest in the beginning. It is the rest that gives the surplus energy and helps to facilitate improvement. Without improvement and surplus energy you cannot increase activity. Instead of increasing activity by doing sofa activities for a longer time and resting less, you can increase moderately challenging activities and do fewer of the less challenging activities. You might spend most of the day doing quiet things like watching TV and listening to the radio, and the day's main activities are doing light yoga for 20 minutes in the afternoon and having a visitor for an hour in the evening. Then, when your body is ready, you could increase the yoga and the visit, and instead do less with the TV and radio. It is not time to increase the most challenging activities until you can do a fair amount of those that are moderately challenging. After quite a while it might be time to reduce the amount of rest. You should only do that when you get as much out of a shorter rest break than you got out of a long one earlier.

When you have severe ME, you usually have many and long rest breaks, and just a few quiet activities. An example could be sitting for ten minutes and resting for half an hour before and after. In that case you can increase the activity level by doing a little more and resting a little less. If you rest for a whole hour, one minute more or less will not make much difference. If you, on the other hand, rest for ten minutes, one minute less can mean you don't get enough rest. Therefore, in some situations, it can be an advantage to increase the activity level without decreasing the rest afterwards. The next time you feel ready to increase your activity level, you can choose to shorten the rest break instead of doing more. Less rest is actually an activity in itself. Sometimes it is better to introduce a whole new activity period instead of lengthening one of the old ones. In that case you must make sure that you get enough rest before and after the new activity period. This can mean that you have to move the other activities around a bit.

UNFAMILIAR ACTIVITIES

When you try an activity that you have not attempted for a while, it is usual to get a small burst of symptoms, even if you start off very carefully. One example of this is when I received an iPod as a birthday gift. The first time I used it I became very tired just choosing a song. However, it quickly became much easier – the next time I tried it, it went much better, and after a week I thought that the iPod was much easier to use than my CD player.

If a symptom burst is caused by an unusual activity, things will improve every time one tries the activity and one will quickly get used to it. But, if the symptom burst is caused by having started the activity too early, the activity will continue to feel especially challenging. This is a warning sign. It shows that you should either engage in the activity for a shorter time or put it off until your condition has improved. The first time one does an activity that needs muscle movements you are very unused to, it is possible you will be a bit stiff and sore, just like healthy people get. If, on the other hand, you get stiff and sore from increasing an activity you already know well, this can be a sign that you are increasing your activity too quickly. When the increase is small enough, you do not usually get stiff and sore.

DIVIDING UP NEW ACTIVITIES

When you start doing activities you have not done for a while, it is useful to have a look at which things the activity is made up of. You can then increase one part at a time before trying to do the whole activity at once.

In the paragraph 'Trips Out of the House' in Chapter 19, 'Social Activities', you can read about how you can increase trips to a café, shops and the cinema. In this paragraph I will use showering as an example. In Figure 4 I have listed the things you do when you shower: sitting, walking, washing, sensations, etc. Looking at this list it is easy to see why showering can be very exhausting if you are very ill and have not done it for a while.

You can start by increasing the activity that seems the least taxing, perhaps sitting. If needed you can recline, starting from horizontal, and increasing the angle gradually. Later you can increase one of the other activities that are necessary. While you are working on this you can get used to the sound of showering by turning on the water in the shower for some seconds while you are on the toilet. It is not time to take a shower until you can do all the component parts of the activity in one day, comfortably and without problems.

Increasing every part of an activity by itself has several advantages. First of all it becomes simpler to evaluate when you are well enough to try out the whole activity. Secondly, the activity will be less of a shock for your body when you are well enough to try the whole activity. You already know how your illness reacts to the different components of the activity. You cannot force your body to be ready for an activity it is too ill for, but by testing each part separately you reduce the risk of relapse from overexertion.

The problem with ME is that the cells' energy production is decreased. You have not simply become unused to doing an activity – it is more complicated than that. It is only possible to increase activity when energy production is improving.

FIGURE 4 – SHOWERING CONSISTS OF THE FOLLOWING PARTS:

- Moving to the bathroom.
- Undressing.
- Coping with the bright light in the bathroom.
- Getting into the shower or bath.
- Sitting/standing long enough to shower.
- Coping with the sound of water and the sensation of water against the skin.
- Washing.
- Coping with the possible smell of the soap.
- Getting out of the shower/bath.
- Putting on a robe or drying yourself.
- Moving back to bed.

AVOID ONE STEP FORWARD AND TWO BACK

"Everything happened in a backwards kind of way – I took two steps forward, then three back, and then two steps forward again! That way I move one step forward, just in a very strange way!" (Shula, AYME Graduates, May 2006.)

The pattern Shula describes is a version of the 'two steps forward and one back pattern'. This pattern is caused by increasing activity too abruptly or too quickly, so that you wear away your surplus, the healing rest, and you end up with a setback. This pattern is unfortunate in several ways. First of all, the setbacks make you more prone to setbacks caused by other occurrences, for example an infection. Many people with ME have experienced getting more infections if they are functioning at the limit of what they can cope with. Also, it is demotivating having to cut back when you are finally able to do a bit more. And, perhaps the most important of all, 'the two steps forward and one back pattern' will most probably mean that you get better more slowly because you are continually spending time getting over the effects of the last increase. Luckily, this pattern is easy to change. You do this by consciously increasing in smaller portions and maybe a bit less often. That way you can accomplish the increases without the backward step. In the long run this can make for a quicker, safer and more stable progress.

AVOID SETTING FIXED GOALS

It is not a good idea to set fixed goals for yourself, such as being capable of a certain activity half a year from now, or that you will increase by a certain amount each week. First of all you get very disappointed if you don't reach your goal. You also risk becoming so absorbed in reaching the goal that you reduce other activities in order to increase the one activity fast enough. You may even overlook warning signs and increase anyway. That last alternative is a sure way of getting a relapse, and actually the quickest way of making sure that you will not reach your goal. It is better to have a goal that is doing what is best for your body, even if this sometimes means that you have to increase more slowly than you would really like. In the long run this is probably the approach that is the most likely to give an effective improvement.

BEWARE OF WARNING SIGNS

The warning signs that show that you should not increase activity can occur at any time during an increasing process. The worst thing you can do in that situation is to continue increasing as though nothing had happened. That is the surest way of going straight into a relapse. It is better to put off the increases as soon as you get an infection, or are subject to a lot of stress or other strains. In these periods your body needs any surplus energy to cope with the strains. When everything has quietened down you are more likely to be able to continue the increases without relapse.

MASKING

In connection with overdoing it you can experience a short-lived masking of symptoms. Masking makes activities that you really know are far too much seemingly go well. The reaction comes after some hours or days in the shape of a strong symptom flaring. Nikki gives this explanation:

> *"Often the bad effects of overexertion don't kick in for one day or two days so I'm resting and thinking, 'well, I did really well and I don't need to pace like this so much anymore,' and then it hits me badly. And no matter how much I think I'm resting, it isn't enough and I keep going downhill. Once I'm back to doing it properly though I get the benefits again, often quite quickly."*

As far as I know, no one has done any research on what causes these delayed reactions. In healthy people exercise leads to the production of endorphins. Endorphins are the body's own pain killers. It is not impossible that the temporary symptom-reducing effect after overexertion in ME patients has to do with endorphins. This might be why the reaction after to overexertion often appears several days later. It is important to be aware that masking of symptoms is a warning sign, not a sign that you are getting better. If you experience masking in connection with increasing activity it is a sign that you have increased too much and should cut back.

IF YOU ARE SCARED OF INCREASING

It is perfectly natural to be worried about doing too much and increasing activity too fast. This is particularly true if you have experienced a few relapses as the result of over-activity. In some people this concern can make them mildly over-cautious. It can help to have a daily routine and also to keep an activity diary. These tools give a better overview of, and control over, your activities. That makes it easier to evaluate whether it is safe to do more. You can read more about routines and diaries in Chapters 6 and 4, respectively. Another tool is to make rules, for instance that you must wait for a certain amount of time between increases no matter how well you feel. Collaborating with a health professional could also help. If your condition is stable and improving slowly, trying out a small increase is not dangerous as long as you listen to your body's signals and cut down again if you begin to feel worse. Even if it turns out that these small increases are too big they do not usually lead to big relapses, just to a few bad days. Remember that activities you are very unaccustomed to can lead to a small symptom flare the first few times you try them. The first increase can feel scary. As you learn more about your limits the scariness usually turns into security and self-confidence.

A TIME OF GREAT CHALLENGES

The time when you are increasing is a period of many challenges. One is often uncertain as to whether it is advisable to increase, or which activities one should choose. One can also become frustrated over the process being so slow, or disappointed by the fact that being able to do a little more wasn't the heaven one thought it would be. At other times it is scary to do something you haven't done for a long time, partly because you are not sure whether you can do it, and partly because it is a long time since you have been in that situation. Thoughts and feelings like this are quite common. It is important to face them instead of sticking your head in the sand. It helps to talk to someone you trust, whether it is family, friends, health professionals or others who have ME. If you choose to talk to others with ME it is easiest to find understanding in someone who is also improving. Those who are in the middle of a relapse may not feel like talking about how difficult it can be when improving. Some of the emotional aspects of pacing are discussed in Chapter 14.

WHEN DOES THE PROCESS OF IMPROVEMENT STOP?

When the process of improvement stops is highly individual. If the process stops long before you are approaching normal functioning level, this could be due to complications. These could be simultaneous ongoing infections, untreated food intolerance or other illnesses. Sometimes the improvement process stops because you are increasing activity too fast.

The Belgian professor Kenny De Meirleir has pointed out that severely ill patients often claim they are well when they are fully out of bed even if they are still unable to work. It is, of course, important to be happy that you are getting better, but you mustn't stop pacing even if you are capable of making dinner yourself. Big changes are difficult to get used to, so in that kind of period you are more prone to doing too much than in other periods. This is also true of the transition from moderate to mild illness when you are trying to increase your participation in a job or in education again. It is also important for people with very mild ME to continue pacing. For one thing this will help to keep you as healthy as possible. For the second, it can prevent relapses, even in people that seem to have recovered fully. It is a comfort that pacing is much simpler when your functioning level is almost normal. Although you may not be among those whose level of functioning is close to normal, you can still enjoy knowing that even a slight improvement in functioning level usually makes pacing considerably simpler.

TASKS

1 Read the list of warning signs that show when you should not increase the activity level and evaluate whether it is safe for you to increase now. It can be very upsetting to realize that you are not well enough to do so, but, instead of despairing, read the other chapters in the book to work out the strategy for pacing that works best for you. That way you will most likely be able to increase later on.

2 If you are ready to increase activity, plan a small and realistic increase. Carry it through and see how it works out.

3 Write a log book of your increases. A list like that is great to have on a bad day when you are feeling that you are having no improvement at all. It is also handy to avoid getting mixed up about when you last increased, and then end up increasing too fast.

SUMMARY OF CHAPTER 8

1. Relapses in ME may have a number of different causes, including overactivity, infections, stress, vaccinations, accidents and other stressors.

2. Those with more severe ME can also have relapses caused by sensory stimulation like sound, light, touch, smell and taste.

3. To stop a relapse you must reduce the level of activity as quickly as possible to a level that does not lead to symptom increase. Make sure to get extra rest.

4. You should have at least one enjoyable activity to look forward to each day, in order to cope with the waiting period until you feel better, but the activity has to be so small that it won't give symptom increase.

5. As the symptoms subside you can slowly increase activity back to the level you had before the relapse. This must be very gradual since an increase that is too quick will lead to another relapse.

CHAPTER 8:

RELAPSES

INTRODUCTION

ME is a fluctuating illness. Relapses are therefore unavoidable. Yet there is a lot you can do both to prevent a relapse and to reduce the severity of the relapses that cannot be avoided. In this chapter I describe the reasons for relapses, the signs that warn you a relapse may be on its way, and how pacing can help to subdue relapses.

In order to minimise or possibly avoid an impending relapse you have to know what causes them. In 1994, the American researcher Fred Friedberg asked a group of patients what the reasons were for relapses they had experienced. The answers listed in Figure 1 are taken from Friedberg's book, *Coping with Chronic Fatigue Syndrome. Nine Things You Can Do*. The list has several weaknesses. The book does not tell us how the figures can be interpreted. For example, it says that 25% of the patients have become worse from vaccinations, but not how many of the patients had actually had a vaccination. Yet the list is still interesting. In some of the reasons for relapse you have a good chance of avoiding them by making changes. If some foods make you worse, you can change your diet and solve that problem. Other things on the list can unfortunately not be changed, for example the weather. If changes in the weather make you worse you cannot change the weather itself, you just have to find ways to live with it. The list shows that the most common reasons for relapses are overexertion, exercise, emotional stress and other infections. Relapses caused by overexertion will be the main theme in this chapter. Before I discuss that I will go through some of the other reasons for relapses.

FIGURE 1 – RELAPSE TRIGGERS RATED BY INDIVIDUALS WITH CFS

RELAPSE TRIGGER	CFS RESPONDENTS (N = 300)
Physical stress (doing too much)	97 %
Exercise	85 %
Emotional stress (upsets)	80 %
Other infections	75 %
Emotional trauma	65 %
Chemical exposure/air pollutants	56 %
Physical trauma	60 %
Humid weather	57 %
Allergens	56 %
Hot weather	47 %
Barometric pressure	45 %
Certain foods	43 %
Cold weather	41 %
Medications	32 %
Vaccinations/immunizations	25 %
Pregnancy	13 %
Birth control pills/oestrogen supplements	9 %

Fred Friedberg, PhD, *Coping With Chronic Fatigue Syndrome*

EMOTIONAL STRESS

It is not always possible to avoid stress or difficult situations. For that reason it is important to be aware that stress management techniques, especially relaxation, can improve the situation. In people with ME it is normal to experience symptom exacerbations from stress, and many doctors, among them Fred Friedberg, recommend that you learn stress management techniques. The relaxation response is the opposite of the stress response. By using relaxation techniques before, during and after stressful situations, you can minimise or avoid a relapse.

Relaxation CDs are widely available from shops that sell CDs, for instance Amazon.com and Play.com. There are also many free downloads and mobile phone apps available. A list of good quality relaxation resources can be found at the back of the book.

OTHER INFECTIONS

You cannot always avoid infections, but certain precautionary measures can help. You can ask family and friends to stay away when they are ill. Good hygiene, especially for your hands, is also important. In some situations using a facemask can stop contagion. In some ME patients repetitive infections can be a sign of overexertion. The following illustrates this: *"When I push myself I get a cold once a month. When I don't push myself I hardly ever get sick."* Acute infections can lead to serious relapses in people with ME. The risk of this can be reduced considerably by making sure to get enough rest in the infection period. Ruth, an experienced ME patient, says that she usually rests intensively as soon as she notices that she is about to get an infection. This usually results in the infection passing quickly and without leading to a relapse.

VACCINATIONS

Vaccinations lead to a strong stimulation of the immune system. According to patient organisations it is, unfortunately, not uncommon for vaccinations to lead to bad relapses in people with ME. Several doctors, among them Dr. Charles Shepherd, recommend that the need for vaccinations is carefully considered. He considers that the influenza vaccination among others is unnecessary and that patients should instead stay at home during epidemics. People with severe ME could and should take steps to try and avoid catching flu. Instead of taking the vaccine themselves, they can ask the people around them to get a vaccination. In some situations it can be necessary to have a tetanus vaccination. One should, though, avoid going on holiday to places where vaccinations are necessary. Luckily there are lots of exciting places in Europe, North America and Australia where it is not necessary to have vaccinations before going.

SENSORY INPUT

There is a reason for relapse that is not mentioned on Friedberg's list. Sound, light, touch, vibrations, smell and taste can worsen symptoms in people with ME. In those who are severely ill, sensory stimuli can give symptoms for several hours after even a short exposure, and a stronger or longer-lasting sensory overload can give long-lasting relapse. In those who are not bed-bound it takes a great deal more before sensory input produces lasting symptoms. Still, this group too can experience strong relapses as the result of lasting noise, like noise from building or road work. In 'Tips for Energy Conservation' you can find advice on how to reduce sensory input. The sensory sensitivities will not necessarily go away with the suggestions mentioned in Chapter 23. However, the problem can usually be managed well enough to avoid a lasting relapse.

WARNING SIGNS

In order to recognise that a relapse is on its way and hopefully stop it from developing into a catastrophe, you have to know which warning signs tell you that the relapse is coming. Many experience a relapse like lightning from a clear sky. Often there may have been warning signs that went unnoticed. When the condition is unstable and the symptom level is high it isn't always easy to see that the bad days have become even worse than before. A high and unstable symptom level is in itself a sign that you are operating at the edge of what you can tolerate and there is a great risk of relapse. You must therefore strive to establish stability and as low a symptom level as possible. How this can be done is described in Chapters 9, 10 and 11. There are, though, other warning signs apart from the unstable condition and a high symptom level. Figure 2 shows a list of warning signs of acute overexertion.

One of the interesting things about the list of warning signs of acute overexertion is that several of them are visible to other people. This means that other people can help by noticing the signs and making sure that you rest in time. The problem is that these are not the first warning signs that show that you are about to do too much; they are signs that show that you have already done far too much and should rest immediately. You should tell family and friends that these symptoms are signs of overexertion. Talkativeness, wiredness and slight hyperactivity are not symptoms people usually connect with ME. People tend to interpret them as signs of wellness, not as signs of what they actually are, namely that you are so overtired that you cannot manage to quieten down. Good communication with the world around you can be of great help here, especially because it is not always easy to notice these symptoms yourself. Others usually notice them first. Figure 3 lists warning signs of bigger relapses.

FIGURE 2 – WARNING SIGNS OF ACUTE OVEREXERTION

- Pallor
- Panda face (red cheeks, white ring around mouth, dark shadows around eyes)
- Sweating
- Noticeably worse balance and coordination
- Slips of the tongue and difficulty finding words
- Pauses in conversation
- Slow movement, thought and speech
- Talkativeness
- Slightly hyperactive (wired)
- Sudden angry outbursts or other types of emotional instability
- Lasting and increasing overstimulation, making it gradually more difficult to both set limits and to rest
- Sore throat
- Acute increase of sleep problems

List is put together by Ingebjørg Midsem Dahl based on patient experiences.

FIGURE 3 – WARNING SIGNS OF BIGGER RELAPSES

- New symptoms
- More and more bad days that gradually get worse
- New or worse food intolerances
- Frequent infections

List is put together by Ingebjørg Midsem Dahl based on patient experiences.

New symptoms are one of the points on the list of warning signs of bigger relapses. New symptoms, though, can also be a sign that you have a completely new illness. It is therefore very important to discuss new symptoms with your doctor to make sure that you haven't contracted some other illnesses that could be treated. This is especially important if increased rest doesn't remove the symptoms fairly quickly.

HOW TO MINIMISE AN APPROACHING RELAPSE

When you notice that a relapse is on its way, or discover that you are in the middle of one, it is very important to immediately reduce activity considerably. If the relapse is caused by something other than overactivity, you should first of all attempt to remove the cause of the relapse, for example to stop eating the food you cannot tolerate. Yet it is still wise to do less for a period because you are more likely to relapse due to overactivity when you are more ill than usual. Many people say: "Yes, I have cut back!"

The question is: Have you cut back enough? What often happens is that you cut back a little, but that you deteriorate even further before you have properly established your new routine. Then you have to cut back some more, and you can go on like this for a long time, maybe even several years. It is better to cut back drastically and stop the relapse, than ending up in a long, drawn-out, downward spiral. Halving all activities can be an efficient way of stopping the relapse. This is a variety of the fifty per cent solution, which was presented in Chapter 1. You should also increase the amount of total rest considerably. If you are among those who do not rest, introducing 4-6 half-hour rests daily will often make the difference. It is, of course, no fun doing far less for a while, but it is much more fun to do less for a period and after that get slowly better, than to do only a little less and perhaps not get better at all. It should be mentioned here that, if at all possible, it is important to introduce at least one enjoyable activity every day. It is not easier to get through a relapse if you deny yourself all the fun. At the same time you must make sure that the pleasant activities are so short that you avoid symptom flares. Otherwise there is a risk that the relapse could get worse.

The techniques needed to stop a relapse are reminiscent of techniques you use to help stabilise your condition. They are described in detail in Chapter 11. The difference is that in a relapse you must often reduce the activity level even more in order to change the way things are developing as quickly as possible. During a relapse you don't need to be worried about reducing the activity level too much. If you do much less for a short period, there is little risk of being harmed by underactivity before you are better again. Underactivity is discussed in Chapter 13. What you must beware of is the danger of doing far too much as soon as you begin to feel a bit better. Many become so over-enthusiastic when they begin to improve that they quickly fall back into old habits and do what they did before the relapse. Then they usually crash right down again and risk getting even more ill than they were during the first relapse.

Increasing activity must always progress gradually, even if you feel that you are back where you were. How you can increase in a safe way is described in Chapter 7. The advice in Chapter 11 is also relevant.

****

Is it really as simple as this – doing little enough for long enough will pull you out of a relapse, and that avoiding overexertion prevents most relapses? Yes, in the main it is that simple. The problem is that it is not simple. It takes a long time to learn pacing and even very experienced patients can miscalculate and end up doing too much. On top of that there is an element of luck. Sometimes everything happens at once and then it isn't always possible to avoid doing too much, no matter how well you plan and how disciplined you are. When that sort of situation arises it is important to remember that relapses are a part of ME. There is no reason to rebuke yourself because you are not perfect. Instead, you should use your energy to do something pleasant that makes it easier to endure the waiting until the relapse is over. When things are at their worst, remember that the relapse will actually pass, even if it takes a long time.

TASKS

1 Which reasons for relapses have you experienced?

2 Have you noticed any of the warning signs before the relapse?

3 Make a plan for what you will do next time you experience warning signs that suggest you are headed for a relapse. Here are some ideas:

- Put off tiring activities such as showering and washing up.

- Put on the answering machine.

- Rest more.

- Cancel appointments.

- Practise relaxation.

- Make and follow a daily routine for especially bad days.

- Make a box with fun cuttings/videos/audio books/ cartoons or the like that can cheer you up on a bad day.

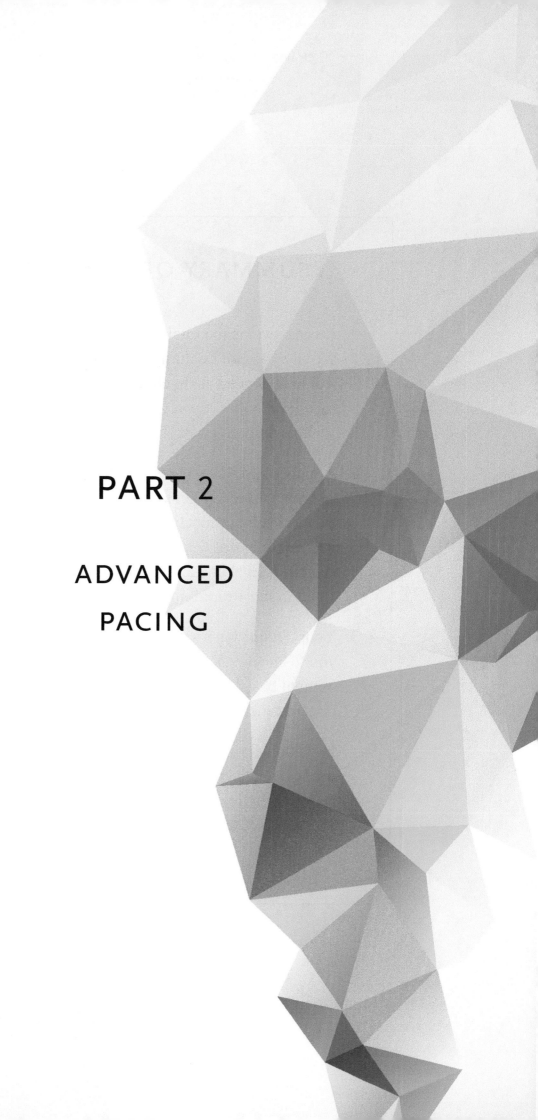

PART 2

ADVANCED

PACING

SUMMARY OF CHAPTER 9

1. A base level is the total accumulated amount of activity you can do during a day without getting worse. It is possible to choose a higher or a lower base level within the region one would consider a suitable amount of activity.

2. A higher base level gives a higher symptom level and you can easily get symptom flares and relapses because you are functioning close to the limit that you can tolerate. A lower base level gives a lower symptom level and a more stable course that can result in more rapid improvement.

3. Your circumstances might make it impossible for you to choose the base level you would prefer. The optimal base level takes your illness, your circumstances and your personality into account.

4. In the long run your illness and circumstances may change, and it can be necessary to reassess and choose a different balance. It is also important to prioritize activities that increase your quality of life, but within the limits of what you can tolerate.

CHAPTER 9:

PACING IN THE SHORT AND LONG TERM

INTRODUCTION

Both healthy people and people with ME can harm themselves by overexerting far beyond their limits. It is also possible to do so little that it is harmful. Between these two extremes there is an area one could call sustainable activity. This area stretches from an activity level that is a bit high without being unhealthy, to a level that is a bit low without being detrimental. The area of sustainable activity is usually a lot lower in people with ME than in healthy people. In this chapter we look at how we can choose an activity level within the secure area. When I use the expressions higher and lower activity level in this chapter I mean higher or lower levels inside the secure area. The consequences of functioning at an activity level that is too high are discussed in most chapters in this book, among others in Chapter 8, 'Relapses'. An activity level that is too low is discussed in Chapter 13, 'Underactivity'.

THE BASE LEVEL OF ACTIVITY

The base level of activity is the total amount of activity you can do in the course of a day without becoming worse. A base level that is so high or so low that it is harmful is not suitable to our purpose and will not be discussed here. Within the area I call the sustainable activity level it is usually possible to choose from several different base levels of activity. Let us have a look at three hypothetical examples.

THREE EXAMPLES

Mary wishes to get the most out of her energy and therefore has a higher base level. She does not stop activities until she begins to get symptoms, but she does still stop quite a while before the illness forces her to. Her rest breaks are mainly used to recover. Since Mary stays so close to the limit she can handle, it does not take much before she gets strong symptom flares. In the course of a year this means a number of smaller relapses. Mary feels ill all the time.

Mona has chosen an intermediate base level. She stops all activities at the first mild warning signs. Her symptom level is therefore markedly lower than Mary's, but Mona does rather less than Mary. Mona has a safety margin. She does not function close to the limit she can manage. Because of that she does not get symptom flares as easily as Mary, and she has far fewer relapses. The symptom level Mona has during her flares is reminiscent of Mary's usual symptoms. Therefore Mona experiences a greater degree of bodily well-being in her daily life.

Martha has a lower base level. She tries to stop all activities before she gets any signals from her body. She therefore usually has no symptoms. When things do not work out as expected and Martha ends up having to do more than she had planned she gets mild symptoms. She seldom has considerable symptom flares. Martha's activity level is far lower than Mary's and also lower than Mona's. Yet Martha feels that the bodily well-being she experiences outweighs the frustration of doing fairly little. Even if Martha is free of symptoms much of the time, she will get strong symptom flares if she overexerts. Just like the others, she would then feel acutely ill. If Martha does much less than usual, she will get symptoms from doing too little, such as general dullness, sluggishness and stiff muscles. She has become good at avoiding this. She uses her body as much as she can, but not more than she can.

LOW SYMPTOM LEVEL IS A RELATIVE CONCEPT

The Mary, Mona and Martha examples are hypothetical and schematic. In reality it is not actually possible for everyone to rest so much that you get a really low symptom level. With severe ME a 'low symptom level' with a low base level means that you have strong symptoms, but that they are a little less awful than they would have been if you had attempted a base level of activity that is a bit higher. In the same way the concepts high and low base level vary according to how ill you are. If you have severe ME, a 'high' activity level will still be low. A low base level in a person with mild ME will lie far higher than a high base level in a person with severe ME. Even if you are among those who get a truly low symptom level by choosing a lower base level of activity, it will usually take some time before the symptom level goes down. Karina, who tells us her story between Chapters 1 and 2, says she had stronger symptoms early on when she was severely ill. Five years later she was almost symptom free as long as she stuck to quiet activities. For the 27-year-old woman who tells her story between Chapters 10 and 11 things moved much more quickly, while for others it will take more time. It is not always enough to use pacing alone. Many need different medical treatments in addition.

CHALLENGES AT DIFFERENT ACTIVITY LEVELS

A higher activity level gives a somewhat higher symptom level, but this can make it easier to remember that you have to break off the activities in time. At a low symptom level it can be very tempting to do too much. However, a lower base level does have an advantage since you have a slightly larger safety margin. If you should make a mistake sometimes, you may well get away with it without it resulting in great consequences. At a higher base level you must be very careful about pacing because it takes so little to overstep your limits. Since there are disadvantages to both a higher and a lower base level some people feel that they may as well choose a lower base level because this gives a quicker improvement in the long run. For others that is not the best solution.

DOES A LOWER BASE LEVEL RESULT IN IMPROVEMENT?

In the short term a lower base level will usually lead to a somewhat lower symptom level, and as a consequence greater physical well-being. In the long run you may also experience an improvement in your functional ability. This has to do with the theory of repairing rest and healing rest, which is described in Chapter 10, 'Two Kinds of Rest'. At a lower base level you usually get more healing rest, and that increases your chances of improvement. According to the theory of repairing rest and healing rest, Mona and Martha would therefore have a better chance of improving, and they would improve more quickly than Mary. In reality there are so many factors at play that you cannot be sure it will work out this way. This, too, is discussed in Chapter 10. There is one aspect that is important to grasp, namely that not all symptoms will necessarily improve. Symptoms that are caused by eating something you cannot tolerate must usually be treated by dietary changes. Other symptoms will have to be medically treated by your doctor. This can happen in connection with symptoms that are caused by active infections. Still, a lower base level can lay the ground for improving in the long run.

DO YOU ACTUALLY HAVE A CHOICE?

In several places in this chapter I have spoken of choosing a lower or a higher base level. This is actually misleading because you do not always have a choice. Sometimes outside factors such as lack of assistance, family obligations or emotional situations result in you not being able to rest as much as you would like. At other times the illness is in a phase where you have no choice but to function at a low base level no matter what you would have preferred. These reasons are real and legitimate, including the emotional reasons for choosing a given activity level. Sometimes it is simply impossible to control life. It can be frustrating, especially if you would like to have a more thorough degree of pacing than it is possible to arrange. It can help to focus on the idea that a perfect pacing strategy, which cannot be carried out, is not actually perfect. This means that the best strategy during some periods is to have a higher base level, while during other periods it will be best to have a lower base level. The important thing is to use our knowledge of the different base levels to adjust the activity level in a better way in daily life.

PACING IN THE LONG RUN

When you have been pacing for a period of time, the routine usually starts slipping so that the base level increases. The result may be that any improvement you may have experienced stops, or starts to go far more slowly. It is natural for the routine to start slipping. No one can manage to stay focused on pacing constantly over a period of many years. Most people with long-term ME are good at pacing themselves, and are skilled at avoiding the dramatic ups and downs that are common early in the illness. Having periods when you do not focus intensely on pacing is not likely to be very harmful as long as you avoid doing so much that you get worse.

CHANGES CAN BE NECESSARY

At times you may find that you need to focus anew and make changes in order to restart improvement, reduce troublesome symptoms, or to deal with a relapse. This is tough, but Nikki, who has had ME for 23 years, points out that you often get quite quick results. What has to be rethought and changed will, of course, differ from one person to another. Here are some suggestions that usually work:

1. A lower base level can reduce symptoms and kick start a gradual improvement, or stop a downhill slide.

2. Greater variation in activities can reduce symptoms that are caused by too similar activities. You can read more about variation in Chapter 3, 'Cognitive Activities'.

3. Shorter activity spells can result in real improvement in symptoms because you stop before you get symptom flares.

4. Taking more rest breaks can give more healing rest and stop deterioration or initiate an improvement.

5. Techniques for energy conservation can give you more leeway in your daily life.

6. A longer time span between increases in activity level, and very small increases can give you a safer and more stable improvement in the long run.

7. More pleasant activities make it easier to avoid sadness and hopelessness. One doesn't necessarily get better quicker by only doing fun things, but you don't necessarily get better quicker by only doing useful work either. The best thing is to find a balance between the activities.

A young woman recently gave me a good example of which beneficial effects you can get out of changing your pacing strategy. She told me that it had occurred to her that she was doing too much mentally and resting too little. When she reduced her mental activity and increased her resting she became markedly better, and she is now better than she has been for over ten years.

SLOW DETERIORATION

Some people with long-term ME get gradually worse, but this happens so slowly that they do not notice it themselves. There are many possible reasons for this, but one possibility could be that they have a base level that is just a tad too high, so that they are being slowly drained of energy. Very slow deterioration (or improvement) may be easier for other people to notice than it is for yourself. If you feel your health status has been at a standstill for a long time it can be a good idea to ask the people around you whether they feel that you are gradually becoming worse. That way you might be able to take steps to hopefully stop the deterioration. You could use some of the suggestions mentioned earlier in this chapter. In the same way you could ask people who understand your illness very well whether they think you are improving because that sort of comment can be quite motivating when your own impression is that your progress is very sluggish. It can be worthwhile, when progress is very slow, to try out some of the suggestions for change in order to see whether that might speed things up a little.

NEEDS CHANGE OVER TIME

Many of those who have been pacing for a long time have said that their needs change as the illness and their circumstances change. When that happens you may find that solutions that worked well previously no longer function as well. Try reading this book again to see if some of the solutions that were not suitable for you earlier might work well now. Perhaps you can develop some of the suggestions so that they are tailored to your needs. When you come across new and improved solutions it is a good idea to share them so that others, too, can benefit from them.

QUALITY OF LIFE

I have underlined the importance of finding pleasant things to do. Finding something you really love doing means a lot when you are pacing in the long run. This could be an old interest that is reminiscent of something you had planned to enjoy if you had not contracted ME, or it could be something new. Perhaps you have to do the activity in an unusual way, but that is not necessarily a disadvantage. I suppose this advice can be summed up like this: Pacing is much easier if you try to live life, but within your limitations. Luckily, pacing often makes it possible to have a life despite ME. It might be a small life, but it will still be your own.

FINAL THOUGHTS

One last thing you should be aware of concerning long-term pacing, is that the illness basically cannot be controlled. We can influence some of the factors that affect the illness, but not all. All we can do is to adjust conditions so that our bodies are as well as possible and hope for the best. Each of us must find a balance where we feel that the effort we make to cope with our situation is worth it. Others have no right to judge the choices we make, because it is not their life. Keep Zoë Williams' words in mind:

> *"...people with ME get criticised a lot. It's incredibly difficult to cope with being so ill and missing out on so much. We're living with a very challenging illness, and just getting by is a 'success'."*

Pacing does not always lead to improvement even when you have a low base level. Yet many patients feel that a lower base level subdues symptoms enough to reduce the amount of time they are acutely ill. You are still left with limitations, but it becomes more like being disabled and less like being really ill all the time. A disability is easier to live with because you can, to a degree, find ways of getting around it. That is not always possible when you are acutely ill.

TASKS

1 What is your base level now?

2 What would be the optimal base level for you now? Take as many circumstances into consideration as possible when you evaluate this.

3 Make changes in your base level if you find it necessary.

SUMMARY OF CHAPTER 10

1. According to the theory of repairing rest and healing rest there are two types of rest in ME.

2. 'Repairing rest' is my name for the rest you take when you have done too much and have to rest to get over it.

3. 'Healing rest' is something you take when you are already rested. Healing rest makes you feel better than you did before the activity.

4. It seems that the more healing rest you get, the better effect you get from pacing. You should try to stop every activity before you get an increase in symptoms. Then all the rests will be healing rest.

5. It is possible to do too little, but most have such a strong wish to do things that doing too little is not a problem.

CHAPTER 10:

TWO KINDS OF REST

INTRODUCTION

"Without rest recovery will not occur." This quotation is from the book, *Living with ME* by Dr. Charles Shepherd.

Are there two types of rest in ME? Over the years I have read innumerable patient stories about pacing. The effect has varied from people with very severe ME who got much better quickly, to people with mild ME who barely had any effect except increased stability. I have also read about more or less every possible combination of different levels of functioning and degrees of improvement, or lack of improvement. The reasons for these differences can be:

- Lack of treatment for infections, food intolerances or other allergies.
- Individual differences in the stubbornness of the illness.
- Differences in support from your surroundings.
- Pure luck.

Yet we cannot ignore the fact that there might be one other factor that plays a role, namely the thoroughness of the pacing.

I made two graphs for a lecture I held the autumn of 1998. These were meant to show the difference between stopping an activity early and continuing until the symptoms become so bad that one is forced to stop. The times on the graph in Figure 1 are only an example. The length of time a person can keep up an activity varies from one person to another. On the line marked with diamonds on Figure 1 you can see that the person starts off with a moderate symptom level of five out of ten. On the other line the squares show when the activity began and ended. There is a strong variation between people when it comes to how long a person can maintain an activity. According to the figure the activity lasted an hour. The triangles show the rest break afterwards. In the beginning of the activity the symptoms remain the same, but after an hour the symptoms were so bad that the person had to break off the activity. Afterwards the person rested for a long enough time for the symptoms to revert to the starting point. The unusually long restitution period seen in ME is well documented. You can read about that in Chapter 22. A young woman once said to me: *"I thought I paced my activities, but in reality I kept going until things stopped by themselves."* That is what Figure 1 shows.

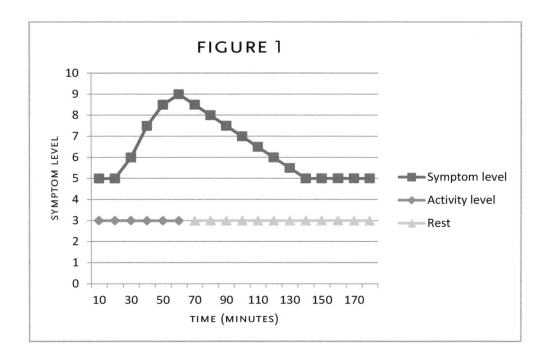

The line marked with diamonds in Figure 2 shows us what happens when the person decides to break off the activity after half an hour. At that point the symptom level has just increased by one step. The result is that the person does not need to rest as long to feel better. After half an hour's rest the person can manage another activity period without the symptom level getting higher and higher throughout the day.

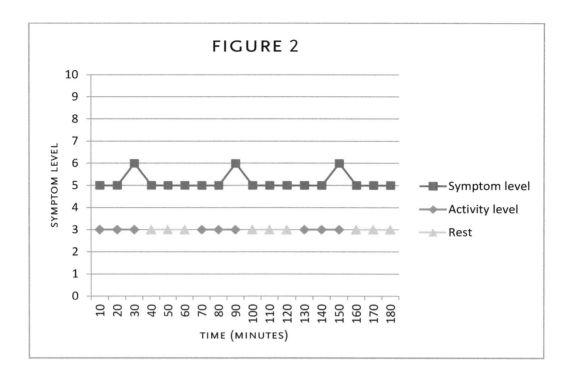

FIGURE 2

People with ME, no matter how severe their condition, report that shorter activities, which do not feel too taxing, aid in keeping symptoms under control.

A while after I had made these diagrams it occurred to me that there was a third possibility. It is inspired by William Collinge. In his book, *Recovering from ME*, he talks about something he calls the 'fifty per cent solution'.

> *"The essence of the fifty per cent solution is that you are spending half the energy you feel is available, and you are investing the other half in your body's healing process. It takes energy to heal. Energy that is spent outwardly is not available inwardly to energize your healing process. You are investing in a savings programme that collects interest."*

This was part of my inspiration when I thought up the third way of doing pacing. What if you broke off the activity before you got any symptoms at all, and rested even if you didn't feel you needed it? The pattern would probably be like Figure 3, namely that the symptoms gradually improved more and more. Here the person breaks off the activity after a quarter of an hour and before the symptoms have increased at all. After 20 minutes rest the person is a bit better. Then the person does another round of 15 minutes that doesn't give symptom increase either and after the next rest period the person feels even a bit better. Notice that the squares and triangles in this graph mark spells of 5 minutes, while those in Figures 1 and 2 marked spells of 10 minutes. In Figure 3 the symptom level goes down from 5 to 4.5 first, and then from 4.5 to 4. This was done so that the improvement would show up on the graph. In reality an improvement would come much more slowly. If the pattern seen on Figure 3 is possible to obtain, it can be used to create a strategy for pacing that may lead to far more efficient improvement than the traditional approach. On this basis I developed the theory of repairing rest and healing rest.

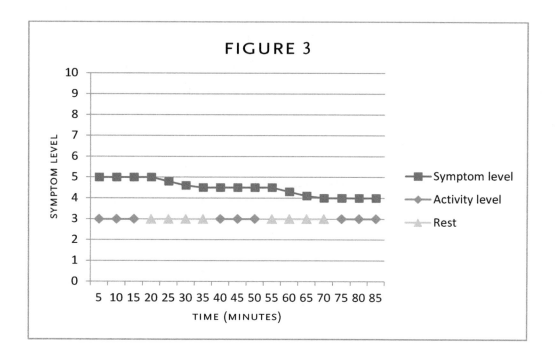

REPAIRING REST

According to the theory of repairing rest and healing rest, repairing rest is the rest you get when you have done too much. Repairing rest is the most common form of rest in ME. More or less everyone with ME knows the sensation of lying on the sofa and feeling the energy slowly returning after having done too much. That is repairing rest. The rest returns us to where we were before the activity which led to symptom increase. This happens quickly, within minutes, hours or days. Repairing rest is an indispensable tool in ME. When a person with ME has done too much it is very important to rest right away, in order to get over the activity as quickly as possible. If you attempt to continue as usual there is a risk of dragging the worsening on for months. Worst case you risk a downward spiral. Repairing rest is only repairing though. To maximise your health you also need healing rest.

HEALING REST

The other type of rest is healing rest. Healing rest is the rest we take when we are already rested. It can bring us a step forward and we get a little better than we were before we began the latest activity. Many people with ME have not yet discovered that healing rest exists. The norm is that we continue with an activity until we feel tired and then we rest until we can manage to do a bit more. Then we start on a new activity. This is the natural way to do things, but this way all the rest breaks are repairing rest and few or none are healing rest. There is no energy left for healing which may hinder improvement, and the rests are likely to be unpleasant due to symptoms. According to the theory of healing rest and repairing rest it is the amount of healing rest that determines how effective the pacing is. If you get just a little healing rest each day, with luck you may see slow improvement in your health.

The good news is that the improvement may be faster if you get a lot of healing rest every day. The prerequisite for this is that there are not too many factors working in the opposite direction, for example active infections, untreated food intolerances, stress, extreme sleep disturbance and lack of treatment for treatable parts of the disease process. In order to get the maximum effect out of the pacing you must stop activities before you get tired and then rest while you still feel that you have the energy to continue. That way all the rest breaks are healing rest and few or none are repairing rest.

THE DIFFICULTIES CONNECTED WITH HEALING REST

There are three things that make healing rest difficult. The first is that you have to rest when you feel ok. That is not natural for most of us. It is boring too. In order to get better it is necessary to learn to rest despite still feeling that you have energy to continue. There are some things that make it easier to learn this. For example, you should teach yourself to enjoy the sensation of well-being during healing rest breaks. Having a lower symptom level is in itself a gain and it is easier getting through the day if you don't feel very ill the whole time. Listening to relaxation tapes during the rest breaks can make it easier to rest because you are doing something. Also it is very important to have several small, pleasant activities in the course of the day. That way there is always something to look forward to when you lie down to rest.

The second thing that makes healing rest difficult is that it takes a long time before it works properly. Often it doesn't seem as though it is working while you are doing it. When doing repairing rest you can often feel that it is doing you good. That is not the way it works with healing rest. Even if you can notice small changes in the course of a few days, it will usually take several months or years to reach appreciable improvement. It is hard to put up with a low activity level for months at a time even if you are good at finding pleasant things to do in between rest breaks. People often become so impatient that they increase their activity level far too quickly. That will often lead to stagnation, or to a relapse. Others give up long before there really has been much improvement. Keeping an activity and symptom diary can make it easier to bear up, because the diary shows the small changes that are easy to overlook in daily life. Two ways to keep an activity and symptom diary are described in Chapter 4.

The third thing that is difficult about healing rest is getting it to function in practice. Life has a way of getting in the way of activity pacing. For people with severe and very severe ME it can be difficult, because they expend much of their energy on absolutely necessary activities like eating. For those with mild and moderate ME, healing rest shouldn't be too difficult to attain as long as they don't have too many other commitments. The problem is that most people have a number of obligations. Lack of practical assistance can force people to do tasks they really aren't well enough to do, such as preparing meals and clearing up. Lively families can take a great deal of energy, particularly if you have small children or you are a single parent. Applications for social services, benefits etc., are often mentioned as a major stress factor that makes it difficult to get enough rest.

Unfortunately, there are no magical solutions, but there are a number of tips and techniques that can make it easier to get enough healing rest. In severe ME it helps to split activities into the smallest portions possible, so that the symptom flares are not greater than necessary. Having some help to relieve the burdens and getting enough assistance is absolutely necessary. It can also help to make sure that you get one or more rest breaks during the day that last long enough to give healing rest.

These tips are just as helpful for people with milder ME. If you are in that group you may also find it helpful to use energy conservation techniques and get practical assistance from the community for things like housework. Good routines can make it easier to live with a lively family. Is there a time of day perhaps when you can organise fixed rest breaks, for example while the children are watching TV? If you are struggling with an application for social services or the like, you might be able to ask for help from a social worker or lawyer, or through a free advocacy organisation. You can find more ideas in Chapter 23, 'Tips on Energy Conservation', and also in Chapter 2, 'Energy Conservation', Chapter 6, 'A Flexible Routine', Chapter 19, 'Social Activities' and finally in Chapter 18, 'Severe ME'.

HEALING REST AS ACTIVE REHABILITATION

There is another technique that makes it easier to put up with healing rest, which is looking at healing rest as active rehabilitation. Even if rest can be looked upon as something passive, there are many opportunities for an active approach to it. I have previously mentioned active experimenting with keeping within one's limits, activity diaries and other tools. In addition, you can actively choose an amount of rest which gives you the best results. There seems to be a link between the amount of healing rest and the speed of any improvement. This can be illustrated with three hypothetical examples. They are derived from the theory on repairing rest and healing rest.

Carl chooses to rest intensively for four weeks. He does this by shortening all activity periods so that none of them make his symptoms worse. He also adds several rest breaks. He gets a lot of healing rest in this period and the symptom level goes down moderately. Four weeks is just an example. Some people would need considerably more time before they notice changes in their symptom level, while others might perhaps notice the effect more quickly. As the symptoms gradually improve a bit, Carl thinks he is much better and can do more. So he increases his activity level quite abruptly. He ends up with an activity level that is a little higher than it was before the rest period. Yet the improvement process stops because he no longer gets healing rest. Carl remains at the same level for months.

Conrad does the same thing and rests intensively for a month, but he is a bit more careful and does not increase activity as abruptly. Conrad decides to increase his activity level only a little bit at a time as he feels a bit better. That way the amount of healing rest remains the same and the gradual improvement continues. This form of improvement is called linear improvement. Linear improvement does not mean totally continuous improvement. In ME there are far too many factors that have an effect on the improvement process for that to be possible. There will always be good days and bad days. Linear improvement must be understood to be a slow improvement process that does not gain speed as time goes by.

Curt also rests intensively for four weeks, but as opposed to Conrad and Carl he does not start to increase activity as soon as he feels better. He waits a bit extra and that way ends up with more healing rest than he had originally. When he begins to increase activity he increases it so slowly that the amount of healing rest continues to rise. This means that, all things being equal, Curt's improvement speed will continue increasing according to the theory of repairing rest and healing rest. You can compare this to letting your money remain in a bank account. That way you get compound interest, and after a time get more and more money on your account. This form of improvement is called exponential improvement (a percentage increase). Exponential improvement is much slower than linear improvement in the beginning. But the exponential improvement moves much more quickly as the increase gets up speed. However, it takes the patience and self-control of a saint to keep up this method!

This is where it can help to think of healing rest as a form of active rehabilitation. It is much easier to persist with a tough setup when you have a clear purpose. At the same time it is not always possible to choose thorough pacing. Sometimes one is in a situation where it is not possible to get as much rest as one would like. Even if you should be so lucky as to have an optimal situation, the way forward will never be straightforward. We are not talking about a 100% stable improvement curve where you get better day by day. Relapses are a part of ME and not all relapses can be avoided. There are also considerable variations in how persistent the illness is. If there are a number of unfavourable factors present at once, thorough pacing may not lead to improvement. Instead, a relapse may become milder than it otherwise would have been, or a downhill spiral could be slowed down. Even though patients' experiences suggest that thorough pacing has a better effect than the less thorough variety, you cannot be sure that pacing alone is enough to produce improvement. Despite these reservations I have read about several people with ME who have gained substantial improvement thanks to systematic use of healing rest. The 27-year-old woman who tells her story right after this chapter is a good example. No matter how much or how little improvement you can gain through the aid of healing rest, it can be easier to stick to healing rest if you think about it as active rehabilitation.

IS IT POSSIBLE TO DO TOO LITTLE?

An important question in this connection is whether it is possible to do too little and rest too much. Theoretically, this is perfectly possible. In the long run you would be harmed by doing too little. At the same time people say that it is difficult to do too little when you have ME. People often have so little practical help that it is impossible to do too little. On top of this most people have such a strong wish to be active that they are emotionally unable to get so much rest that it becomes harmful. Experienced patients say that the body sends out signals saying that it wishes for more activity if you rest a bit too much, and that these signals turn up long before you get symptoms that show that you actually have been harmed by too much rest. You can read more about this in Chapter 13, 'Underactivity'.

****

A young woman with very severe ME told me that she had experienced a drastic reduction in her symptom level by resting even when she didn't need it. As the years went by her activity level improved too. Today she is out of bed and well enough to go out. As I said in the introduction to this chapter the theory of repairing rest and healing rest is so new that no research has yet been done on it. Therefore, we have no research based proof of the theory, but experience suggests that it is correct. If this young woman is a representative example, then there is a lot to suggest that healing rest can be an important tool in managing ME.

TASKS

1 Make changes in your activity and rest pattern so that you get as much healing rest as possible and as little repairing rest. This will usually mean shorter activity periods and longer, and more, rest breaks.

2 Learn at least one relaxation technique so that you get as deep a rest as possible.

3 Think of, and use, at least two strategies that make it easier to live with your new rehabilitation programme. The strategies may be emotional or practical.

WOMAN, 27 YEARS OF AGE

Yes, pacing is fantastic! It has really changed my life. Since we last spoke things have only moved in one direction, up, and it doesn't look like it's going to stop any time soon. It feels so quiet and good inside my body because there's no war going on in there any longer. It can't be described, and I am so thankful for pacing being so effective once I got into the swing of it and my body got the adjustments it needed. It is a way of life. Either you do it or you don't. Because it only works if you are consistent and don't lie to yourself and say, "I will probably not get sick if I do this or that..." and so on.

More or less every day is now a symptom-free day. The only thing I cannot manage to pace away is the feeling of not being well, but the rest of the symptoms are kept at bay. I only have symptom increases a few times per week, and that is usually a light cognitive deficiency that disappears with 5-10 minutes rest. For my body it has been a big change to go from having a strong symptom increase several times a day to just having them in a light form a few times a week.

I take things very easy – I'm strict about a maximum 10 minutes' activity to 20 minutes' rest. For a long time I rested in bed with ear plugs, lights off and the whole package, but my body doesn't need such intense rest anymore – now I can rest in a chair instead. This might be because my base level is higher. I can also say that I don't have any practical help at home now, just help to buy groceries once a week. This was my own choice.

I can now manage, with strict pacing, to do all the daily things. It is amazing all the things you can manage to get done by pacing yourself through the day. Some activities are heavier work than others, so I only do them for a few minutes at a time, like emptying the dishwasher or hanging laundry up to dry. I don't get tired or sick, since I stop in good time before that happens. It has also become easy to keep doing this, since the whole thing has become a routine. I don't have to consciously think about not being active for too long, it has become automatic. I've been on a few trips out lately and they went splendidly – it didn't make me ill at all, not even slightly tired. I am very careful because I'm scared of being hit by a setback, but I listen to my body and it tells me that it's ok. For years I got severe muscle pain from going out, but that's all gone now. I haven't experienced that since I started pacing... I didn't think it was possible to go out without getting sicker, but pacing taught me differently.

The difference between going out today compared to before, is that I steal as much rest as I can while I'm out. I zone out for a few minutes, empty my head, breathe deeply and relax my entire body. I do this often, and I am not 'tuned in' the whole time. By that I mean that I don't talk a lot, am not energetic, extrovert, etc., but instead take things veeeeery easy. I also use my aids: ear plugs and sunglasses.

I love my ear plugs – I even use them in the shower and now have a totally different experience when showering. I don't leave the shower like a wreck anymore. I also went to the cinema last week, with a pillow and hot water bottle, comfy clothes and ear plugs. The people sitting around me must have thought I was about to move in, but so what! I enjoyed myself and left the cinema feeling well, and not even tired in my little finger. I haven't been to the cinema for several years, so it was very nice to have the opportunity to do it again.

I have been given a new body and a whole new life. During the last few months there hasn't been a single awful day. It is almost unreal. This is the most effective treatment I have ever tried! I really believe in it!

You might say that pacing is about giving away activities and giving up your freedom, living under strict rule and unable to do a lot of things you would like to, but the truth is that for me this has been the key to freedom! I am better than I have been in several years. I have had a stable and good condition for 4 months. That has never happened before! I get more and more freedom every day that goes by and the energy level just increases, because the body is getting what it needs to get better, pacing and rest.

Yes, I was indoors for 7 months and just concentrated on doing everything the right way and build up energy from scratch, but that was a small price to pay for all the things I am left with now! And most of us that don't pace, crash quite often and then are forced to lie in bed and not do anything. And it is much more comfortable to choose, for a time, to reduce energy use in order to gain all the good things that turn up after a while. So why not choose the alternative that is the least unpleasant and the least destructive for both the future and the body?

In any case, I now, for the first time in a long time, look with pleasure at what the future will bring, because there are a lot of good things coming and that is thanks to pacing.

Learning pacing has been a challenge for me, also personally. It gives me a pleasant feeling of managing my daily life and situation that I will carry with me in my future life. I would not be without this experience. It gives hope for the future and a factual and concrete plan. Nothing in life is as important as living, and moving forward. Even if things sometimes move forward with tiny steps.

This text is presented here with her consent.

SUMMARY OF CHAPTER 11

1. ME can be split into three stages according to how aggressive the illness is.

2. The unstable stage is characterised by a high symptom level, very unstable activity level and high illness activity in the body.

3. The stabilising stage: At the stabilising stage the symptoms are far more stable, the activity level is more stable and the symptoms are on their way down, but the activity level cannot be increased.

4. The remission stage: At the remission stage the symptom level is low. One becomes gradually better and can increase the activity level slowly.

5. To improve the chances of moving from the unstable stage to the stabilising stage, one must stabilise activity at a low level which does not give symptom increase. In order to move from the stabilising stage to the remission stage you must hold the activity level stable even when you begin to feel a little better. In the remission stage you must not increase too quickly or abruptly because this will lead to relapse.

CHAPTER 11:

THREE STAGES — THREE MANAGEMENT STRATEGIES

INTRODUCTION

Several attempts have been made to split ME into stages. Most of these stage models are either about the length of the illness or about functional ability. Several stage models take it for granted that persons with ME, who have a high functional ability, have a low symptom level and perhaps even that they are improving. Similarly, they assume that people who have a moderate level of functioning also have a moderate symptom level. In reality, it's a lot more nuanced. For example, it is quite possible to have a high activity level yet at the same time a high symptom level because the person is heading for a relapse. It is also possible to be severely ill, but to have a moderate symptom level because one is improving.

The English paediatrician Alan Franklin's stage model differs from other models. It describes the degree of illness activity in the body, that is, how aggressive the ME is at any given time. The degree of illness activity is decided by symptom intensity and stability.

Franklin split ME into three stages: the toxic stage, the stabilising stage, and the remission stage. At the toxic stage you have a high symptom level and the illness is very unstable. At the stabilising stage the symptom level is lower and the illness is considerably more stable. At the remission stage you have a low symptom level and get better so quickly that you can increase the activity level gradually. The stages are not connected to any given functional level. It is therefore fully possible to have a relatively low level of functioning, yet be at the remission stage, or be at the toxic stage, even if one has a high functional level. The interesting thing about Franklin's stage theory is that it can be combined with the theory on repairing rest and healing rest. That way it can be used to choose the right strategy for pacing based on which stage you are at. By choosing the right strategy for pacing you can contribute to reducing illness activity. That way you may get better faster than if you had paced your activities at random. In the following section I describe how this can be done.

FIRST STAGE — THE UNSTABLE STAGE

The stage that I have chosen to call the unstable stage Franklin called 'The toxic stage'. At the unstable stage both the symptom level and the activity level are unstable. The symptom level is high, and you feel ill all the time. According to Franklin, rest is absolutely necessary at this stage, just as in the acute phase of all other illnesses. He stresses that the acute phase in ME often lasts much longer than in other illnesses, and that one returns to the acute phase when in a relapse. Since all forms of exercise lead to worsening at the unstable stage, Franklin feels the activity level should be reduced drastically.

This is sensible if you see it in the light of the theory of repairing rest and healing rest, which you can read about in Chapter 10. According to this theory it is a surplus of rest that leads to improvement. In order to get a surplus, it is usually necessary to reduce your activity.

The goal for pacing at the unstable stage is to stabilise the condition. This can often be achieved by reducing the activity level to a level that does not lead to symptom increase during the day or from day to day. The reason for this is that days with more activity use up energy and provoke severe symptoms. By lowering the activity level to a level that does not lead to symptom increase the body gets the opportunity to start healing. With a bit of luck the symptoms will gradually stabilise. At the unstable stage, many find it difficult to know which activity level they should aim for, since the symptoms go up and down all the time. In that situation the activity diary is an important aid. It is much easier to find out how much you can tolerate when you know exactly how much you do on a good, medium and bad day.

Figure 1 shows how unstable the activity level of a patient at the unstable stage can be. The graph has been made from a 30-day activity diary.

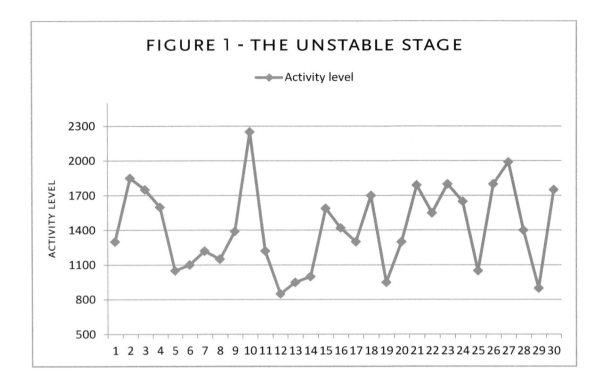

The rule of thumb is: If you stabilise your activity at the level of the highest peaks on the graph you will become gradually more ill. That is because the highest peaks show the days when you overdo it. If you head for the level between the highest point and the lowest on the graph your condition will stabilise, but probably not improve. In other words you will stay static. If you do approximately the same amount every day as you do on bad day, your condition will not only stabilise, it also stands a good chance of gradually improving. The explanation can be found in the theory of repairing rest and healing rest.

At a medium level you will typically get quite a bit of repairing rest and not much healing rest. Your improvement speed will therefore be quite low. Maybe you will not improve at all, especially if there are several other unfortunate factors in the picture at the same time. On the other hand, if you stick to what you can manage on a bad day, even when you are having a good day, you will get quite a lot of healing rest and will hopefully gradually improve. Again this depends on how many other factors are pushing you in the opposite direction. Total stability is difficult to reach in ME since many factors affect your condition at any given time. ME is by definition a variable illness. By stabilising the activity level, your condition will usually become more stable than if you do not.

Most people find it very hard to reduce the activity level. In the beginning, it is therefore important to reduce the level enough to start getting a bit better. Your symptom level will then go down, which is encouraging and motivating and makes pacing more endurable. It is also important to think of the low activity level as something you do to get better. It is an intermediate phase, not a permanent change. In addition you must make sure you do some enjoyable things in your activity periods.

Many people say that the greatest challenge in pacing is keeping the activity level low long enough to get better, instead of becoming too enthusiastic and doing too much too soon. Yet it is a common worry that doing less for a time is harmful. Very long-lasting inactivity can be harmful, but in the unstable period the body needs to recover. In that situation a lower activity level will usually give quicker improvement, and many find they get better so quickly that the inactivity does not last long enough to be harmful. Yet it does take time to get better. If you are worried about doing too little you should talk to a physiotherapist. Inactivity is discussed in Chapter 13.

The time it takes to stabilise your condition varies from person to person. The unstable stage can last for several years. This is especially so if you have to wait for a long time to get a diagnosis, if you are advised to push yourself, or if you don't get enough assistance and support. When you start learning pacing it will take time to get used to the technique and to become familiar with your limits. You don't, therefore, suddenly become stable as soon as you start trying to pace your activities. It is not unusual for it to take several months to really get acquainted with your limits. If you are among those who find it difficult to learn pacing, it can help to ask others for their advice, a professional or a patients' group. You can read more about this in Chapter 1.

Please note that overactivity is not the only cause of instability in ME. Other common causes include food intolerances, viral reactivation and anxiety. When there are several causes of instability present at the same time, it can be difficult to see a pattern and identify the causes. Because the limits of most people with ME are so strict, it can be difficult to stay within them. For this reason, overactivity is almost always among the causes of instability, so stabilising the activity level is nearly always a good place to start. Once the activity level is stable, it will be easier to identify the other causes. However, sometimes the need to stabilise other causes is so pressing that another cause has to be prioritized first. Use your best judgement and get professional help if necessary. The more causes of instability that are dealt with, the more stable the illness will become.

THE SECOND STAGE — THE STABILISING STAGE

At the stabilising stage you find that the illness is more stable and that you may be very, very slowly improving. Franklin points out that it is important to be extremely careful because any form of overactivity will, at this point, lead to relapse to the first stage. The goal for pacing at the stabilising stage is to keep the activity level stable while the symptom level simultaneously goes down. This is often challenging because it is natural to start doing more the moment you feel a bit better. This, though, is not a good idea. If you increase as soon as you feel you have the strength to do a bit more, the amount of healing rest remains constant and slight. This means improvement will continue to be slow. If you keep the activity level stable, even if you feel a bit better, the amount of healing rest will increase. Therefore, the improvement will probably speed up. This also leaves you a security margin that can prevent many of the small relapses.

A flexible daily routine makes it considerably simpler to keep the activity level stable. The activity diary, too, is a good aid. First of all it makes it possible to keep an eye on whether you are actually managing to keep the activity level stable. Secondly, you get to enjoy the sight of your symptom level gradually decreasing. Take a look at an example of this in Figure 2. The symptom level, measured on a scale from 0 to 10, has been drawn on the same graph that shows the activity level.

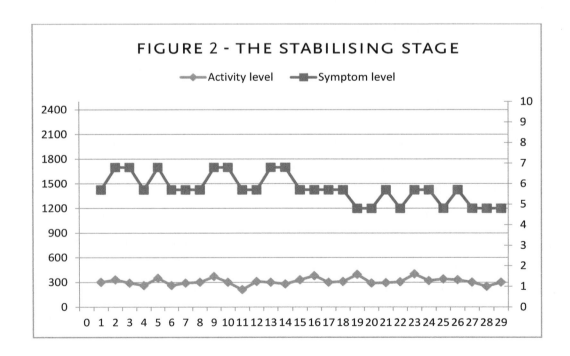

It is much easier to put up with pacing when you can see from your diary both that you are managing to do the pacing, and some of the early signs that your plan is actually giving results. That also makes it easier to believe that this will work out in the end. Since it takes time to experience improvement in ME, it is very important to have some small, pleasant activities to look forward to, so that you can endure the waiting time. It is also important to hang on to the thought that even if things move very slowly to begin with, it does not mean that they will continue as slowly the whole time. This goes for all ME patients at all levels of functioning. Pacing is a very tough rehabilitation technique so you need all the aids you can get.

The time the stabilising stage lasts varies considerably. The norm is that stabilising takes a number of months. Most people try to stabilise their activity level approximately at the level they have on an average day. Some patient stories suggest that the process can speed up if you stabilise the activities at a lower level, that is, below the level you have on a bad day. This makes sense according to the theory of repairing rest and healing rest. When you lower the activity level even more you get more healing rest. Then the body has more energy to heal itself. The young woman who shared her experiences with pacing just before the start of this chapter, had had ME for ten years and never been stable earlier. When she started doing thorough pacing she attained not only stability, but also substantial improvement in six months. Things do not always move as quickly as they did for this woman, especially if you have severe ME. Franklin points out that one can remain at this stage for years. Still, this young woman's story shows that it does not always take many years to reach a higher level of functioning.

If you find that you remain for a long time at the stabilising stage without any sign of improvement, it could be a sign of two things. The first possibility is that you get too little healing rest. The ME researcher Fred Friedberg suggested that you can try to reduce you activity level and then increase very gradually. I would like to add that you should postpone the increasing part until you begin to actually see improvement. As Franklin points out, increasing the activity level too early will land you with a relapse. Another possibility is that improvement is hindered by other factors like food intolerances, infections or stress. A closer description of these unfortunate factors and what can be done about them, can be found in the chapter on relapses, Chapter 8. When pacing has little effect it is especially useful to reduce other unfortunate factors. Be aware, though, that the job of reducing unfortunate factors must not demand more energy than you have.

THE THIRD STAGE — THE REMISSION STAGE

Remission means reduction in force or degree. This characterises the remission stage. The illness has diminished but is not gone. According to Franklin the improvement is obvious at this point. You can increase both physical and mental activities gradually. Noticeable improvement does not mean that a patient gets steadily better day by day. That is usually quite unrealistic. Noticeable improvement means that you are in an upward moving spiral where there is a small, but noticeable difference between how your condition is now compared to how it was a few weeks ago. You can increase your activity every few weeks, or every few days if you are very lucky, and can hold on to the increases over time. When improvement is so slow that you have to look back many months to see any improvement, it means that you are at the stabilising stage, not the remission stage. Figure 3 shows a graph belonging to a person at the remission stage. The dots do not represent days, they represent monthly averages. The graph covers a full year and the person's average activity level increases by approximately 23% from January to December, so we are looking at a slow but clear improvement.

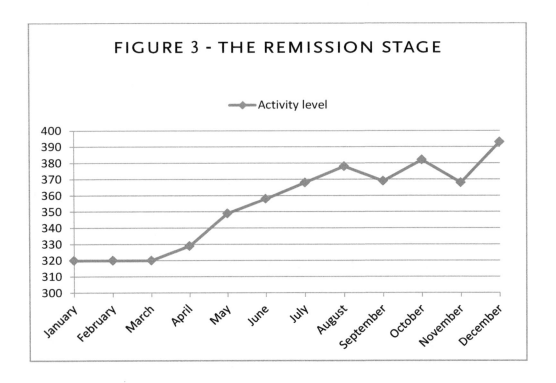

The greatest challenge at the remission stage is to increase slowly enough. When you feel a little better, it is very easy to think that you can do a lot more. The problem is that abrupt increases eat up your healing rest. Many people with ME have discovered that too abrupt, or too quick, an increase leads to relapse or stops the improvement. Patients also report that you have a better chance of hanging on to your improvement if you increase your activity level slowly. Franklin, too, points out that improvement is slow. The increasing phase demands self-discipline, especially in the beginning when the increases are small and one's eagerness to get better quickly is great. Merete Sparre, a Norwegian physiotherapist, points out:

> *"Discipline must mainly be used to hold back when the desire for activity appears in order to avoid relapse, subsequently to find exactly the right dose of daily activity, and also to learn to rest."*

Discipline must not be used to force increases in the activity level. That will only lead to relapse. In the improvement phase it is important not to get the idea that it is the increase that leads to improvement. In reality it is the other way around. It is the pacing that leads to improvement. The improvement then leads to the ability to increase gradually. Once the improvement phase is well established the process of improvement may quicken. In order to make this happen you have to increase activity so slowly that the amount of healing rest gradually increases. At the same time there may be a few negative factors like infections present. In Chapter 7 you can read about how to increase your activity level in a safe way when your body is ready. Franklin emphasises the importance of the patient controlling the improvement process. Increasing the activity level must not be dictated by others.

There is one thing that Franklin does not discuss, which I consider important to include, and that is that the remission stage does not last forever. At some point improvement will stop. This might be a sort of fourth stage where one is stable again, though at a higher level. Follow up studies, among others those done by Dr. David Bell, show that many patients get to be much better than they were at their worst, but that only a few reach a fully normal level of functioning. In a talk by Merete Sparre in 2007 she states:

> *"Many reach a point where they can live without symptoms much of the time, but at a considerably lower level of functioning than they had before. And although there are those who get worse, I permit myself, when speaking to a new patient for the first time, to say, with conviction, that almost everyone with ME gets better."*

I, too, have read of people who have experienced that the illness settles down if they do little enough and are not burdened by other factors. The moment these patients try to do as much as a healthy person can, the symptoms quickly return. It seems that pacing can play a part in keeping the illness in check, but that pacing cannot remove the ME. Pacing is management, not a cure, perhaps in the same way that management of Type 2 Diabetes cannot cure the illness itself.

Even if you have been stable for a long time (including being at a high level) there is unfortunately no guarantee that you will remain stable. Twenty years after the ME epidemic in Lyndonville in the state of New York, David Bell did a follow up study of the children who fell ill during the epidemic. The study showed that even people who had been improving for years may begin to get gradually more ill. Personally, I have many friends who have had ME for 15-30 years. A number of these relapsed some years ago. Luckily, a large number of them are now on their way back up, and some are even better than they have been for the last ten years. They have benefitted from management techniques like pacing and dietary changes. Some have also had medical treatment, but that is something not everyone has access to. Bell's research, the experiences of my friends, and the experiences of people who have sent in letters and articles to the magazines of patient groups, all suggest that both improvement and aggravation can occur at any time during the illness. I have also read about people who got ME again after seemingly having been completely well for years.

In the book *Learning to Live with Chronic Fatigue Syndrome*, Edmund Blair Bolles writes:

> *"Even after you have fully recovered from your CFS, you should pace yourself so that you work at about one point below your maximum level. That is, if you rate your fatigue level at six* [out of 10 possible, where 10 is lots of energy (Author's note)] *work as if it were five. That way, you will always have the energy to meet any sudden demands and will still be able to face the next day. Many people are repelled by the idea of 'giving less than 100 per cent'. It seems counter to everything they have been taught. Sergeants in the military, athletic coaches and corporate presidents all urge their people to give 110 per cent and to 'play through the pain'. But the price of this approach is a short career. If you give more that you can, all too soon you will be giving less than you could have. In his book on acting, the great English performer Laurence Olivier*

advises actors never to perform at the maximum because the signs of strain become visible. Always keep something in reserve. That philosophy led Olivier to sixty years of stardom. Pace yourself, pace yourself."

Strategies for pacing based on Franklin's model can be summed up as:

First stage: reduction of the activity level, to a level that does not give symptom increase, in order to attain stability.

Second stage: Stable level of activity while the symptom level goes down.

Third stage: Gradual increase of the activity level without symptom increase.

This management plan turns pacing into an active rehabilitation technique, not just a bothersome way to avoid relapse.

TASKS

1 Find out which of Franklin's three stages you are at. If you are in doubt, assume that you are at the unstable stage.

2 Plan a strategy for pacing that suits the stage you are at. Use the other chapters in this book as aids.

SUMMARY OF CHAPTER 12

1. A reduced sense of exhaustion can occur in persons who have had ME for a long time, even without improvement in the illness. Then it is important to use other symptoms than exhaustion to evaluate how much you can do. Use the small signals.

2. Mental overstimulation, a form of overexcitement, can occur as a result of mental overexertion. Overstimulation can make it difficult to stop activities in time and to rest enough mentally. It helps to stop activities before you feel overstimulated and to learn deep mental rest.

3. Some people experience local loss of functional ability, that is some body parts are weakened considerably more than others. This can occur as a result of overexertion. Here, too, pacing can give a clear improvement of the functioning, but this can take a long time.

CHAPTER 12:

CHALLENGES IN PACING

INTRODUCTION

Pacing involves a rather large number of challenges. In this chapter we will look at three challenges which have not been discussed much in the other chapters of the book. Mental overstimulation and a reduced feeling of exhaustion are symptoms that make it considerably more difficult to pace your activities. Reduced functional ability in certain body parts is also a challenge, since many people feel that it needs very accurate pacing to improve the functioning.

MENTAL OVERSTIMULATION

Many healthy people have felt so exhausted after a long day that they cannot unwind. They try to rest but their head grinds on all on its own. Not many people know that this is a very common problem in ME. The problem is called mental overstimulation. Mental overstimulation has not been discussed much in ME literature and only lately have we begun to see much attention paid to the subject. Experienced patients, though, have discussed this problem for a time, and this section builds on their experiences. Overstimulation shows up in several ways:

- being talkative
- a feeling of being 'wired', or speeded up
- a slight sensation of being 'high' that makes it difficult to stop an activity
- short periods of hyperactivity followed by symptom flaring
- difficulty with stopping one's thoughts during rest breaks and activity periods
- difficulty sleeping
- flushing

Most people with ME have experienced this when they are trying to sleep at night, but overstimulation can also be a problem in the daytime, especially for those who are severely ill. Overstimulation in this group can occur during minimal activity, like thinking for a moment, saying a sentence, or experiencing short-lasting sensory input. It often worsens during the course of the day. It is common for people with ME to think that overstimulation is caused by too much adrenaline, even though this has not been scientifically documented. Some people with very severe ME have found that overstimulation can spiral into a panic attack, but it is perfectly possible to be very overstimulated without having the physical symptoms that one can get from a great release of adrenaline. It is natural to presume that overstimulation may be caused by disturbances in the brain's signal systems. Research has not explained this phenomenon yet. Emily Collingridge advises that people should attempt to remain calm when they are overstimulated, because panicking will only make the symptoms worse. It is worth noting that overstimulation in itself has nothing to do with anxiety. However, nervousness or anxiety may aggravate it because this will increase the energy expenditure and the overstimulation will get worse the more energy consuming the activity is. Similarly, the racing mind you get may aggravate anxiety if you already have it. Still, I know several people who have had severe overstimulation without a trace of anxiety.

Overstimulation is a symptom of overactivity, just as pain, exhaustion and concentration problems are. The most important way to reduce it is to stop activities as quickly as possible. You should also learn deep mental rest. Emily Collingridge also underlines the importance of this. She writes that some people find overstimulation so uncomfortable that they stop resting, but this just makes the problem worse. It can be useful to listen to CDs with relaxation exercises when you need to still your head. It also helps to find out what kind of thinking you feel is the least tiring. If you, for example, find it very tiring to think in words when you are overstimulated, you can carefully force yourself to think in quiet, still pictures. After that you can think of one body part at a time, and in the end your brain may become so calm that you can manage not to think at all.

Overstimulation can make it very difficult to switch off and tune out or even to pace activities at all. This is not down to a lack of self-control, it is caused by physiological disturbances that are part of the illness process. You might compare it to how difficult it is to relax one's muscles when one is in severe pain. Yet it is important to work on learning to switch off as well as possible, so that you gradually become less overstimulated. In persons with severe ME, learning to switch off can make the difference between getting better or not. An example of this is described in Chapter 18, 'Severe ME'. Since the people around you often read talkativeness and hyperactivity as signs of health, and not of overstimulation, it is important that you explain to them how overstimulation works. That way those near you can help you to rest in time and so help you manage your illness more effectively. Even extreme overstimulation can in time become considerably better by using pacing techniques.

REDUCED FEELING OF EXHAUSTION

People who have had ME for a long time sometimes feel that the sensation of exhaustion lessens. In some the other symptoms remain unchanged. Others say that the other symptoms also feel different. The big problem is that it is the feeling of exhaustion that people usually use as a measure of how much they are able to do. Without the exhaustion it is very easy to overrate how much you are capable of doing. This can make it really difficult to decide how much activity you can tolerate. Some people end up going from one relapse to another even though they were stable earlier. On top of this people say that they are now capable of pushing through symptoms that they could not push through when they could feel strong exhaustion. The feeling of being very ill can be intense even though the exhaustion is gone. The feeling of illness, though, is usually a symptom of gross overexertion, not an early warning sign. When the feeling of exhaustion is limited it becomes far more important than before to attempt to stop before getting a symptom flare. It becomes even more important to learn to use other symptoms than exhaustion to take your bearing.

You must not overlook the small signals. It is especially important to keep an eye on your blood circulation. Many people with ME find that poor circulation is a sign of overexertion. You should therefore stop all activities before your circulation gets worse, and rest until it is a step better than it was before the activity. Poor blood circulation can be felt, among other ways, as a tingling sensation or a cold feeling in all or parts of the body. When it becomes so poor that you notice it you have already done too much, and it can be easier therefore to do some concrete experiments to find out where your limits are. You can stop after a certain number of minutes so that you are sure to stop before the warning signs arrive. Experimentation is discussed in Chapter 1.

Another useful tool is learning to enjoy the feeling of well-being that comes with thorough pacing instead of feeling that you must do something every time you feel able to.

Learning to live with a reduced feeling of exhaustion can seem like having to learn to live with ME all over again. The process of learning by experience while one becomes re-acquainted with your body's new signals can be frustrating. Yet it is still fully possible to gain stability and improvement in the long run.

LOCAL LOSS OF FUNCTIONING

Some patients experience a far greater loss of functioning in some body parts than in others. This is more common among people with severe ME, but it can also occur in people with moderate ME. Loss of function in people with moderate ME usually becomes apparent in that the 'bad'" (that is those that seem more affected than others) parts of the body are weaker, more painful and have less stamina than the rest of the body. Persons with more severe ME can experience total loss of their ability to function. You can lose the use of arms or legs, your voice, become too weak to open your eyes, or lose the ability to manage certain thought processes.

This kind of function loss can occur as the result of overexertion. Ruth's story is an example of this. She says her ME started after an intense period of studying for British secondary school exams. All the subjects she took required lots of writing, and this was before it was common to use a computer at school. After four months of illness she started the next school year with a heavy schedule. She says:

> "After one term I was unable to write half an A4 without intense pain lasting into the next day."

The next few years Ruth continued trying to go to school because her doctor refused to give her sick leave. It took three years before she was diagnosed and another two before she got any advice on how to manage her illness. By then she was very ill. She continues:

> "To this day I still have pain in my right arm that prevents me writing an A4 page. If I write infrequently, then I can do so with minimal pain in small amounts 200-300 words. I avoid writing

large amounts at all costs. Typing using Dragon is a suggested alternative, but with swollen glands that also has its limits. Certainly not a viable alternative to work or study. In my experience, overuse of my right arm has left me with a disabling level of pain for twenty years to date."

Many people with ME have learned that this sort of function loss can improve with rest, but my own experience and that of others suggest that it takes healing rest. Repairing rest is not enough. If you attempt to increase consciously (that is, try to train a body part), you will usually slow down or impede improvement. Amy, who has had severe ME for many years, says this about loss of functioning:

"I don't know if anyone has done research on this, but I know that if I continue using my right arm to write, brush my teeth, etc., it gets worse the more I use it. In the end I get to a point where it is so painful and weak, and I lose the ability to grip things. But if I rest it and use it less, for example by doing things with my left arm, it will gradually improve and I can at least use my right arm for some few things. It has taken a long time to get to the stage where I can use it more. Forcing it all the time brought me to a point where I couldn't use it at all. It is only possible to heal it by resting... When people say that not using a part of the body leads to problems/atrophy, I usually overlook it when it comes to ME. All I know is that resting it and not using it, means that I actually can use that part of the body more in the course of the day/week, than if I had continued to use it."

Many have had the same experience as Amy, that is that a 'bad' part of the body just gets worse if you force it to function. 'Nikki', a young woman who has had ME for many years, agrees with Amy. She writes: *"I definitely have to rest a body part when I have pressed it too hard. To continue trying to train it just leads to more waiting time before I can use it again, and then it can only be used well inside its limits."* In addition, I, myself, have seen that if I use the healthiest parts of the body a lot, this can have a negative effect on the worst parts, even if they haven't been used. Philippa, an experienced patient, has experienced something similar. She writes: *"If I overuse any muscle in my body at all, all the other muscles get weaker. So if I have a bad cough my chest muscles get weaker, and so do my arms and legs, etc."* It seems as though one has a total amount of energy that can be distributed to the different body parts. In order to make the worst parts of the body better, you must avoid using the better body parts so much that nothing is left to heal the worst bits. In other words it can be a good idea to choose a relatively low base level of total activity. You can read more about this in Chapter 9, 'Pacing in the Short and Long Term'.

So, it seems that it is healing rest that brings back the functional ability that has been lost. With enough rest and assistance the ability to function will improve on its own. It can, though, take a long time, sometimes, worst case, it can take years. When the ability to function begins to come back, spontaneous increases will be enough. Spontaneous increases are small, almost imperceptible increases that turn up on their own as you begin to get better. Examples of this could be that you shift a bit, stretch a little, or unconsciously continue an activity a moment longer than before. Many people have learned that attempts at conscious increases at an early stage can slow down improvement and lead to serious relapses. You can only increase your activity consciously when the ability to move the body part has returned and improvement is well underway. This also applies when you have lost the ability to move your whole body.

It is unclear whether everyone with ME can regain functional ability in the worst body parts through healing rest. Nor is it certain that the body part will regain full functional ability. In any case, many ME patients have seen that healing rest can make an important positive difference.

****

CONCLUSION

The three pacing challenges discussed in this chapter have caused problems for a number of people with ME. Much of the reason for this has been the almost total lack of information on these subjects, so that people have had to find solutions by themselves. Hopefully this chapter will help make this easier.

TASKS

1 Which challenges have you experienced with pacing?

2 Have you had any of those described in this chapter?

3 Which solutions and coping strategies do you use today in order to tackle these challenges?

4 Are there areas where you would like to find even more solutions? Use this book as an inspiration to develop some that are suitable for you.

SUMMARY OF CHAPTER 13

1. Repairing rest, which is the rest that brings us back to where we were before doing too much, is not underactivity.

2. The experiences of ME patients suggest that repairing rest cannot be overdosed. Healing rest, which is the extra rest you take when you are already rested, can, in theory, be overdosed.

3. Despite this, patients' experiences show that underactivity is uncommon. Most people have such a strong desire to be active that the big challenge is to get enough rest, not to get enough activity.

4. Substantial loss of muscle mass and other symptoms of long-lasting underactivity are infrequent in ME, and this is supported by research. Patients say that they can tell when their body needs more movement than it gets, and that it is easy to increase the activity level at need.

5. People who have had a stable activity level for a longer period say that periods of lower activity than usual can result in feeling dull and sluggish. A small increase in activity level makes these symptoms of underactivity quickly disappear.

6. If you are afraid to increase your activity level because you might overdo it, there are strategies that can help you.

CHAPTER 13:

UNDERACTIVITY

INTRODUCTION

An important question in connection with pacing is whether it is possible to do too little and rest too much, and, if so, how you can tell if the activity level is getting too low. This is what we will take a closer look at in this chapter. In connection with writing this chapter I collected the experiences of about twenty people with ME in Norway and Great Britain. This comes on top of the more than several hundred patient stories I have read in the magazines of patient groups from several countries during the last twenty years.

WORSENING OF SYMPTOMS WHILE RESTING

Sometimes, people with ME, who are not experienced in living with the illness, say that resting makes them feel more ill. In some cases the reason could be that the person has been wrongly diagnosed and has an illness that actually makes one feel worse from resting. At other times it is a question of people thinking they feel worse because they are resting, when the truth is that they feel worse because they have done too much before the rest break.

Mette, who has moderate ME, says:

> *"When I have a longer, relatively good period (weeks and maybe a few months) I can manage to do a bit too much every day without any particularly big crash. Until I crash totally. This is a sort of accumulation of overactivity that can turn up after a while. Furthermore, after such a period of overactivity, it can be difficult to rest well on a bad day because the symptoms are so much stronger and more numerous, and lying still is a challenge because of symptoms like sensory sensitivities, body pain, malaise, breathing difficulty etc. This can be helped by finding something*

that distracts me from the symptoms, like small doses of movement from time to time, such as getting up and moving around a bit, watch TV for a bit, or listen to an audio book. It could be that some patients misinterpret these symptoms of overexertion to mean that they get worse from resting and taking care of the body – that the whole thing instead actually is a need for a little movement/activity to mask the great discomfort. My experience, now I come to think of it, is that this discomfort/symptom-increase gradually subsides day by day with proper rest, and thereafter comes down to 'normal' level again after the rest period."

When you are active, you get distracted from symptoms. When resting you notice the symptoms more clearly. Experienced patients say that even though the beginning of a rest period can be tough, resting eases the symptoms after a while.

REPAIRING REST

In Chapter 10, 'Two Types of Rest', I explained that there are two types of rest in ME, repairing rest and healing rest. Repairing rest is the rest we take when we have overdone it. It brings us back to where we were before doing too much. Everyone with ME who I have spoken to agrees that repairing rest is absolutely necessary in order to get over overexertion. Without rest you cannot recover, and you need more rest the greater the overexertion has been. Most have never experienced negative reactions to repairing rest, except that it can be boring. One person went so far as to say that it had never occurred to her that underactivity could be possible, and that she did not even know the word. Heidi stated categorically:

"If all underactivity is restorative rest, it is not underactivity."

HEALING REST

Healing rest is extra rest that you take when you are already rested. There is a risk of underactivity here. Yet most of those I have spoken to say that they have not experienced negative consequences here either. The reason seems to be that most people have such a strong need to be in activity that they in reality are not capable of resting long enough for it to do any harm. When people begin to notice the effect of healing rest, that is, when the symptoms begin to lessen, they begin to feel bored. Many also feel guilty and think they have to catch up with all the things they haven't been able to do while they rested. The point is that our need for activity functions as a natural protection from underactivity. At the same time this natural protection hinders people from getting better because they don't get enough healing rest.

SYMPTOMS OF MUSCULAR UNDERACTIVITY

The natural urge for activity is not the only protection against underactivity. The body also sends out other signals. People who have experienced underactivity agree that these symptoms are easy to recognise. For example, one woman told me that she needed several rest breaks at regular intervals during the day, but that she could feel it when her body needed more movement if she had rested too much.

Zoë Williams, who has severe ME, says:

> "No, I cannot say that I have experienced negative effects of underactivity. When my health has improved I've noticed, for example, specific muscle pain in my back from sitting up more than I was used to, which I suppose was 'deconditioning'. However, this was very easy to identify, nothing like the toxic ME impact of having done too much, and so I was happy to see it as a natural part of the process of improvement. It didn't make me think my health was going downhill, it just seemed natural that my muscles would complain."

A feeling of stiffness, pain and tight muscles can be a sign that you have not used your muscles quite enough. One patient who experienced this said that her experience was that it took very little increase in activity to get rid of symptoms like these and that the symptoms got better quickly. If muscle symptoms are caused by overactivity, attempts to increase activity will often give a strong increase in many other symptoms, among others the feeling of being ill. The muscle function will also usually get worse with use. These signs can aid you in discerning the difference between symptoms that are caused by overactivity and those caused by underactivity.

CONTRACTURES

Inactivity over a very long period brings symptoms that are considerably more serious than the symptoms mentioned earlier. Tendons and muscles can become so tight that joints cannot straighten out fully. This is called a contracture. Contractures tend to sneak up over a longer period and can be discovered at an early stage if one keeps an eye on how mobile a joint is. I have only heard of contractures in connection with severe ME. The most frequent form is that the ankle gets stiffer so that it is no longer possible to stand with your foot flat on the floor. This is called foot drop. A Danish woman who developed this when bedbound, told me that it only took small, regular amounts of stretching in order to straighten out her feet when she began to get better. Others tell me that tiny amounts of movement within the body's limits are often enough to prevent contractures. For that reason there are many ME patients who never develop contractures even though they are bedbound for years.

Be aware that some people with ME get acute muscle contractions in connection with overexertion. This is likely a form of spasm rather than contractures. A Norwegian girl got spasms in her legs and back muscles after an acute overexertion and couldn't stretch out her legs. A British girl got the same symptoms in both her arms and legs. While she was severely ill these lasted for up to several months, but when she got better they occurred acutely if she overexerted and disappeared overnight. Others get the same symptoms in their fingers. When spasms occur as a result of overactivity it is absolutely necessary that any stretching is done within the body's limits so that the spasms do not get worse. Stretching is not necessarily a good solution. You should experiment cautiously until you find the solution that works best for you.

LOSS OF MUSCLE MASS

Another result of long-term inactivity is losing muscle mass. In the eighties a number of studies of muscle specimens from ME patients were done. The book, *The Clinical and Scientific Basis of ME/CFS*, by Byron Hyde summed up the research done by Peter and Wilhelmina Behan, who did several such studies. According to this summary there were a number of abnormal findings, but in the majority of patients the specimens showed no sign of the type of muscle loss that occurs with underactivity. The conclusion was therefore that most ME patients use their muscles as much as they can tolerate.

When I had been bedbound for five years I had visibly thinner legs. At the same time I was well enough to move a bit more than earlier. A minimal increase in physical activity quickly gave a visible increase in muscle mass. My physiotherapist confirmed that both the muscle mass and activity level increased as my health improved, and therefore my physiotherapist was not worried at all about the loss of muscle mass.

Be aware that overactivity can also lead to loss of muscle mass. In the article, *Reporting of Harms Associated with Graded Exercise therapy in ME/CFS*, Tom Kindlon quotes an Irish patient who had filled in a questionnaire on graded exercise therapy. She wrote the following about her experiences with four months of physiotherapy: *"When I went to the hospital I could walk 100 yards, feed, wash and dress myself. When I left I could not weight bear at all, had no leg muscles to speak of, and needed two people to transfer me on and off the toilet and in and out of bed."* In the cases where loss of muscle mass occurs as a result of overactivity, it is absolutely necessary to stop the overactivity so that the muscle loss does not get worse. Both yourself and any professional health care workers must respect the body's limits and choose measures that you feel give you a good effect.

GENERAL UNDERACTIVITY

In addition to muscular underactivity there is yet another type of underactivity in ME, namely 'general underactivity'. This sort of underactivity is not common either. Only very few of the persons I have spoken to have experienced this type. What they have in common is that they say that if they do considerably less than they can without getting worse, they become dull and sluggish and run into problems falling asleep at night. The symptoms they mention are restlessness, passivity and problems with sleep.

Sarah says:

> *"When I was say around 40% level or higher I did find if I did less than I was capable of in a day it wasn't helpful – my brain/body wouldn't be tired enough to sleep that night."*

Heidi says:

"For me, getting to know my body's reactions well has made all the difference. When my condition kept swinging up and down, I 'landed' after periods of high activity. I got worse because I had been too active, and it became absolutely necessary to have a long period of rest. After a time I noticed that my body was strengthened by the rest, that is, first it got much worse, then gradually better, but after that, my body got dull, passive, restless and sleepless. I can quite easily tell the difference between 'landing' and becoming dull and passive because of underactivity. When I told the psychologist who helped me learn pacing about the underactivity symptoms, he said – but Heidi, you are not bad, or lazy and definitely not depressed (which I feared) when you feel that way. You have 'unemployment sickness' – and most healthy people would experience much the same if they were kept in passivity for a shorter period (weeks, a few months)."

All of those asked agreed that it is necessary to do less than usual on bad days. The symptoms of underactivity appear only if you rest far more than you need. One person pointed out that this phenomenon did not occur for the first years of the illness, but only later when the illness had become more stable. This is not particularly odd. When the illness is unstable, frequent overexertions will mean that one needs a lot of rest, and almost all of it will be repairing rest. To the degree one gets extra rest this will not be enough to go from healing rest to underactivity. In the book, *Mindfulness for Health*, by Vidyamala Burch and Danny Penman, they recommend that you place yourself at a level that is 80% of what you can manage without getting symptoms so that you have some safety margin. If you are capable of doing an activity for 10 minutes without getting symptoms then you should stop after 8 minutes. As long as you increase gradually when you begin to get better, this strategy should hinder healing rest from turning into underactivity.

Sarah, who was quoted earlier, points out that she has not experienced general underactivity after she became severely ill. At the moment she is so ill that she simply cannot manage to rest too much. The great majority of those who have severe ME have never experienced underactivity. Philippa, who has had severe ME for many years, says:

"I find that a day of doing less than usual or even having total bed rest for a day/a few days, gives my health a real boost. It certainly doesn't make the ME worse. If I rest completely for more than three days, a little bit of deconditioning occurs but it is easily reversed again. Overactivity on the other hand, is always very dangerous and detrimental."

In severe ME the risk of overactivity is a far greater danger than the risk of underactivity, because daily activities like eating and toileting in themselves may represent overactivity. Nor in milder degrees of the illness is it common to do too little. This is partly because the majority have a strong need to be active, and partly because the majority have responsibilities that in themselves cover all or most of the need for activity. Also, the body sends out clear signals when it wants more activity. Once you have learned to recognise the signals, it is relatively simple to avoid doing too little.

WHEN THE BODY'S SIGNALS ARE DISTORTED

Is it possible that the body's signals can sometimes get distorted, so that people do not notice that they do too little? In the course of the last twenty years I have read about a small handful of people with ME who did too little for a period of some months as a result of severe depression or anxiety on top of ME. In these cases it seemed as though the feeling of depression or fear was so strong that it covered up the body's signals about the person doing too little. At the same time the symptoms of anxiety and depression were so obvious that all the patients were given help before the body had time to be damaged by the low activity level. Some of you who read this will probably wonder if it is possible to be so depressed or anxious without being aware of it yourself. This is not something one needs to worry about. Such serious anxiety and depression is obvious both to the person and to those around them. Nor do all those who have depression or anxiety on top of ME necessarily become underactive. I have spoken to several people who have a tendency to do too much despite the fact that they have anxiety or depression and are undergoing treatment. You can read more about depression and pacing in Chapter 14, 'Accepting Pacing'. Some persons with ME who have experienced setbacks caused by overactivity develop a mild degree of being overly careful and are frightened of increasing their activity level. This is quite natural. This kind of anxiety does not have to turn into underactivity. In Chapter 7, 'Improvement and

Increasing Activity' you can find tips on managing fear of relapses.

In addition to straightforward depression and anxiety, I've recently become aware of another potential cause of general underactivity in ME. Research has shown that some people with ME underproduce beta endorphins. Endorphins are opioids (morphine-like substances) which act as the body's natural pain killers. In large amounts, these will cause people to feel high, like you would when taking significant doses of morphine. However, if the endorphin level is too low, people will experience withdrawal symptoms, which include depression, irritability, fatigue, pain and sensory sensitivities. In other words, a low endorphin level would make a person with ME feel more ill than the disturbances in the cells' energy production would warrant. This, in turn, could result in underactivity. Since most people have a tendency to do too much, a mild deficiency in endorphins probably would not cause underactivity. However, severe deficiency could cause underactivity, particularly if the person is also anxious and depressed and happens to be in a situation where underactivity is possible.

Low endorphin levels are potentially treatable with a drug called naltrexone. Naltrexone is an opioid antagonist (morphine blocker), which is normally used in the treatment of substance abuse. When used in tiny doses, it stimulates endorphin production. In theory, naltrexone could therefore be used to treat underactivity caused by the body's signals being distorted by a low endorphin level.

I am aware of five people with ME who have tried low-dose naltrexone. Two had no effect whatsoever, and two others experienced small improvement. The fifth person experienced drastic improvement. This person had a number of symptoms suggestive of a low endorphin level, including significant depression. Despite years of slow improvement, he was reluctant to increase physical activity. He did not normally leave the house, but on the rare occasion when he had to, this did not lead to overexertion. When the low-dose naltrexone lowered his symptom level, this man happily began increasing his physical activity level steadily without psychological treatment, and he actually became quite hooked on exercise. His depression improved very significantly. It seems likely that this man's reluctance to increase activity was caused by his body sending out too strong signals of discomfort because of a low endorphin level and that the low-dose naltrexone corrected this. Endorphins do have a slight immune modulating effect, and this man may well have had an immune dysfunction, which responded particularly well to this change. However, the main effect of naltrexone is symptomatic.

As mentioned above, I am aware of four other people who have also tried low-dose naltrexone. I know three of these people quite well. What they have in common is that they all operate close to their upper energy limit and have frequent small setbacks because of overactivity. None of them are depressed. They simply do not show signs of a significantly low endorphin level and certainly no signs of underactivity. This probably explains why they did not experience significant improvement from the low-dose naltrexone.

Please note that increasing the endorphin level when it is already normal or high could be counterproductive. It could distort the body's signalling system, just as much as a low endorphin level would, but in the opposite way. It could cause patients to feel less ill than they actually are. The challenges of living with a high endorphin level are discussed in Chapter 12, 'Challenges in Pacing', in the paragraph 'Reduced feeling of exhaustion', and in Chapter 21, 'Pacing of Movement', in the paragraph 'Warning Signs'.

SYMPTOMS OF RECOVERY

One of the things that turned up in connection with the work on this chapter was that symptoms which occur during rest are not necessarily a sign of resting too much or having done too much before resting. Heidi, who has moderate ME, says:

> "I would like to add that that I can get symptom flares during healing rest. I have used a lot of yoga, meditation and relaxation techniques (usually all at once) and this is something that I have had to learn. It takes time to learn to rest and relax properly. When the body is ill and in a state of stress, it is difficult to quieten down totally. Now that I feel I am quite good at relaxation, there are times when I experience pretty strong symptom flaring during and after healing rest. It is almost as though the body is working hard when it gets that relaxed. I often get a sore throat and the flu-like feeling. It passes very quickly and I feel better all day and often several days afterwards."

The symptoms Heidi describes, such as sore throat, are probably a sign of immune activation. When an activation like that is followed by a clear improvement, it is a good sign.

My own experience confirms that symptoms that occur during rest can be signs of improvement. Before, my body was cold and clammy most of the time, but when I used deep rest it gradually warmed up. After a while two things occurred. First I began to sweat a great deal. Then I felt a deep pain in my muscles that was worse at the places where I usually had most pain. In the beginning I thought that these symptoms meant that I had rested too much, but after a while I discovered that the longer I could stand the pain and sweating, the better I felt afterwards. The pain was probably caused by my blood vessels expanding because of deep relaxation. Perhaps this can be compared to the pain you get when the blood comes back to a foot that has become numb because you have been sitting on it. By using deep rest systematically my health gradually improved and the sweating and the pain also got better as time went by. So when symptoms turn up during rest it is not always a question of them all being signs of resting too much.

****

All our experience suggests that overactivity in ME is a far greater problem and danger than underactivity. The most important thing that has become clear during my work on this chapter is that people with ME get signals from their body both when they do too much and when they do too little, and that it is not difficult to feel the difference between the two types of signals. In the few cases where anxiety or depression become so strong that underactivity can become a problem, professional help can hinder underactivity from lasting so long that it becomes damaging. For most people with ME, learning to recognise the body's signals can be the key to finding the right balance so that you avoid both over- and underactivity.

Experience suggests that having enough information, and learning management, can help prevent most cases of both damaging overactivity and damaging underactivity.

TASKS

1 Have you experienced symptoms of underactivity and, if so, which?

2 In which situations have the symptoms of underactivity occurred? Make a plan to avoid such situations.

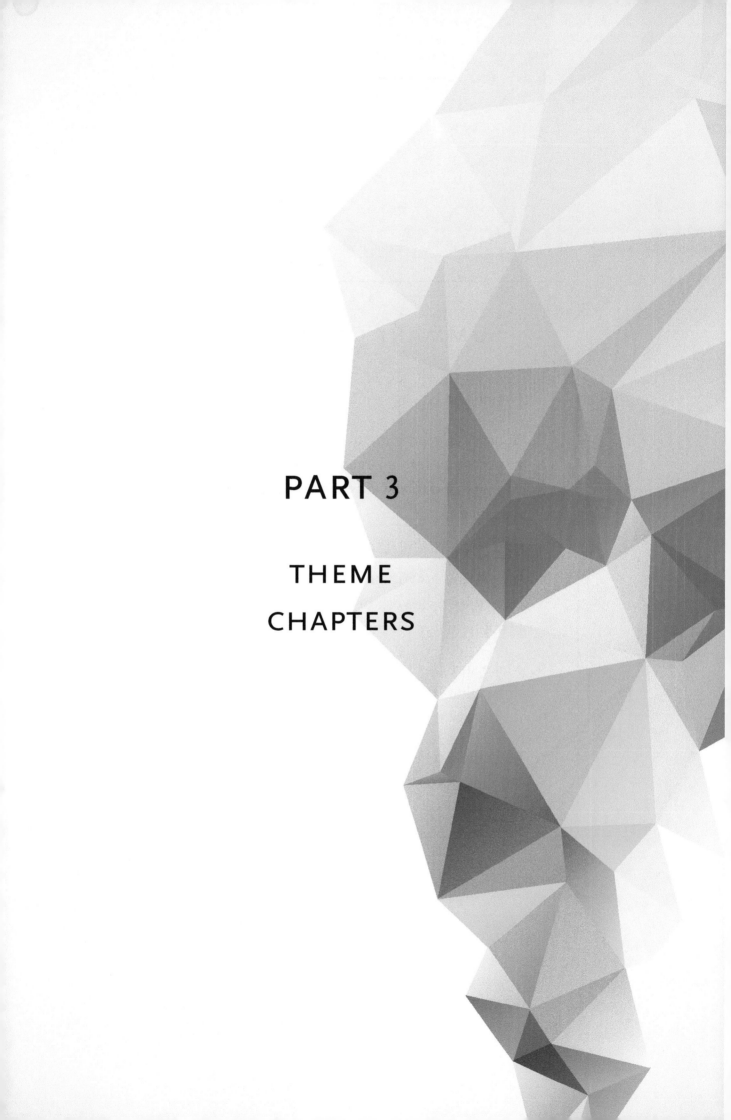

PART 3

THEME
CHAPTERS

SUMMARY OF CHAPTER 14

1. Pacing can be very tough emotionally.

2. In order to get pacing to work for you it is important to find a strategy that is suited to your situation and to reward yourself when you have managed it.

3. The fact that pacing works is not a sign that it is the patient's own fault that they are ill. ME is not caused by overwork or overtraining, and the patient is not to blame for their illness.

4. Make sure that there is a balance between the things that drain you of energy emotionally and things that charge your emotional batteries.

5. It can help to read books on management of the emotional aspects of chronic illness.

CHAPTER 14:

ACCEPTING PACING

INTRODUCTION

One of the most difficult things about pacing is accepting the method. It is not fun to have to limit your activity level over time, nor to have to take rest breaks or do activities in very different ways from everyone else. This chapter is about the thoughts and feelings that are common among people who do pacing and how you can think in order to manage carrying out the technique.

GETTING STARTED

An important point is that in the beginning pacing is all about experimenting. It usually takes several weeks or months before you are so well acquainted with your own limits that you can avoid symptom flares. This does not mean that pacing doesn't work, nor does it mean that you are bad at it. This is just the way things work when you are trying things out and learning from your mistakes. Also, when the condition has stabilised it still takes time (and luck) before improvement sets in properly.

In order to keep up your motivation it can be useful to make lists of things one is good at and things that have improved. This could be lists of situations where you feel pacing works well, of symptoms that are better or have disappeared, things in your life that are good, things you have learned after you became ill, and which increases you may have made when it comes to your activity level. Then you can use the lists as an encouragement when you are feeling frustrated and stuck. That way you avoid giving up too early because you think pacing doesn't work.

If pacing is very difficult, you might have to adjust it to suit your situation in life better. A woman named Ruth told me she had a routine with fixed rest breaks in the daytime, but that it is more difficult in the evening when her boyfriend is visiting. She said: *"It is the overall picture that is the important thing."* There is no reason to blame yourself if you find that there are situations or times of the day when it is difficult to pace activities perfectly. Instead, you can do it Ruth's way and plan your programme so that you get enough rest at other times of the day. That way you can make sure that the overall picture is balanced.

Even if you find good solutions there will be times when you find pacing a pain. Then it might be that it is not the pacing itself that is the problem.

Sarah says:

> "When I started pacing I found I really struggled to accept that all spontaneity had evaporated from my life. The breakthrough came when I realised this wasn't down to pacing, but because of my ME. Pacing is a tool, a way of coping, and to be honest it is just common sense. Yes, it is hard doing things little and often, but it is better than not doing them at all."

STOPPING BEFORE YOU CRASH

Of course it is not fun to have to stop in the middle of a pleasant activity. On the other hand it is not a pleasant experience to feel very ill after going on with something for too long either.

Nikki says:

> "Sometimes it's absolutely infuriating to stop midway through something you love, and sometimes I don't stop. I'll go on until I've overdone it and I can't see any more to read, or my muscles have stopped working and spasm and I drop things, or I'm in agony. Sometimes I'd get distracted reading and not notice until I passed out. Each time it helps remind me that I don't have to always follow the pacing but that I will have to pay for it at some point. Maybe not that minute but some time down the line. When I try to pace I'll be able to go back to something sooner than if I do it until it's caused me serious problems and I can't touch whatever it was again for days or weeks and everything else has been affected too."

If you push yourself to do a lot one day and then need several days to recuperate, you are probably overestimating how much you can do. Overall, one would normally be able to do more in total by spreading it out more evenly.

Sarah says:

> *"It is impossible to 'control' ME, but I did find it empowering to be able to handle things better once pacing levelled out the whole 'boom and bust' pattern."*

If you insist on continuing with activities that you are actually too ill to do, you will quickly become so ill that you cannot manage the activity at all, and it takes time to recover again. If, instead, you dare to take a break where you pace your activities very carefully, you will usually get slowly better and gradually be able to reintroduce the lost activities. You will not necessarily have to give up an activity all together either. Often energy conservation techniques and short spells make it possible to take part to one degree or another.

NOT A QUICK FIX

It will take time before you feel any noticeable change in the symptom level even though the improvement process has begun. Claire Wade explains:

> *"Pacing isn't a quick fix; it's a way of life, like healthy eating. You can't just do it for a few weeks and expect it to be a miracle cure; you have to see it as a way of life. Boring, frustrating and awful at times; but the benefits come in the long run."*

ADJUSTING ACTIVITIES

Amy says that she has to split things up in order to get anything done, but even when one is forced to, it can be very frustrating to have to stop in the middle of an activity. Practical tips on how to split things up are described in Chapter 3.

Claire has also felt the frustration of having to divide things into little bits:

> *"I learnt to do smaller activities, like one sticker on a card or making a tiny pair of earrings, so that I had something complete at the end. I had a lot of short quick activities and then one or two longer ones to keep working on."*

If you have the option of choosing the size of a project yourself it is important to be realistic. It is easier to get a positive experience out of using a week or two on a birthday card, than using a year or two on making a photo album. At other times you are forced to divide a big job into little bits. Then it helps if you try to enjoy the process and be pleased with every new little goal you have reached, instead of getting stressed by not having finished the project yet. Make a list of the little goals because it is gratifying to be able to tick off one after the other.

TACKLING REST

Rest can be a challenge. Some people use activity to distract themselves from painful thoughts. In *ME – en sykdom i tiden* (Nowegiean for 'ME – an illness in our time') by Sidsel Kreyberg, she quotes a young woman with ME:

> *"The hours before I fall asleep are the darkest and loneliest of the day. So I stay awake until I collapse."*

Amy, too, feels that resting can be tough. She writes: *"This is a hard one, sometimes if I really get into it, I find resting is quite enjoyable but other times it's just so tedious."* Yes, resting is boring, but it's a very necessary part of getting better from ME. It is important to focus on the fact that resting keeps symptoms at a minimum and reduces the risk of relapse.

Short and frequent rest breaks are less boring than few and long ones. *"I find the 50/10 or (for me) 40/20 minute split of activity/rest also worked really well. I'm now doing longer rests with longer gaps in between"*, says Victoria. People with severe ME usually need more rest than this, but for this group, too, spreading activities sparsely throughout the day is useful. If you are not used to resting, you can increase the amount of rest gradually.

Claire says:

> *"Start small, just ten minutes at a time and then build up by two minutes per rest. That's what I have done in the past. It sounds silly; but it's much easier to cope with."*

Relaxation techniques can make rest breaks less boring, and at the same time make the rest deeper and more effective. Amy points out that very low energy activities, like cloud watching or daydreaming, can be restful.

Nikki agrees:

> *"I found it much easier to rest once I realised I just needed to find interesting things to think about instead; an imaginary world to inhabit, or playing games in your head are all good. Having somewhere nice to rest with pictures helps too, or thinking of something enjoyable you're going to get to do after resting. Learning not to think about topics that are upsetting and noticing when you start thinking about them and moving on to something else is also important. There's no point going over and over things you can't change. All it can do is make you unhappy."*

FRUSTRATION

Several people have pointed out that frustration over not being able to do much gets a lot worse if you push yourself, while the frustration lessens a lot in periods when you have a good balance between rest and activity.

Zoë Williams says:

> *"It is so frustrating when I do too much. I try to stretch my limits, and I end up fighting with the illness. When I stay within my restrictions, the illness behaves better and I can think that I am tackling it."*

Nikki says:

> *"A problem I do have is patches where I feel like I have cabin fever from being stuck inside so long and not seeing people. It gets very frustrating. Sometimes, the temptation just to give up on my pacing and really blow my energy on something gets really bad.*
>
> *"The nearer I get to being able to do something, I think the harder it gets not being able to do it. That just out of reach but theoretically possible feeling is so much harder than a longing for something so out of reach it's become almost an abstract. However well I normally deal with things there are days where I just have to acknowledge I am going to be frustrated, angry and upset because I am in this position and that it is a normal and acceptable response*

to feel this way in my situation and I should just accept that and it'll pass again. It helps to share this with friends who understand and feel the same way. Because knowing I'm not alone in this is comforting and makes it easier to deal with for some reason."

UNCERTAINTY

Another thing that can be frustrating is the uncertainty of not knowing if or when you might be better.

Nikki says:

> *"I think it would be easier if I knew that I will continue to get better, and that I will be well enough to manage certain things at a certain time in the future, if I stick to what has worked in the past. But the uncertainty in this dumb illness and the unexpected relapses make planning almost impossible. I have great plans and accept that they may never materialise, but I have to take small steps in the right direction and hope for the best. Also, I have some small activities I can finish in one go, and then I can be satisfied because I have started on something and managed to do it."*

OTHER PEOPLE

Often people with ME do not want to be different and stand out from the crowd. This might be because they are afraid of being misunderstood.

Nikki says:

> *"I'd let people presume I could manage the same and then had to deal with the consequences later which is harder. Better to get it out in the open to begin with before they make presumptions about you."*

ME is an almost invisible illness, which often leads to misunderstandings and disbelief. This sort of disbelief is not only an ME-phenomenon, and it is common in all illnesses that do not show. You should be aware that misunderstandings can get worse if you attempt to act as though you are well. That gives people the impression that that you are probably not really as sick as you claim, or that it is all in your imagination. Arriving late, leaving early, taking rest breaks, using aids, etc., can lead to greater understanding. I experienced a great deal of disbelief when I was a child, which made me quite scared of my healthcare professionals. After I became bedbound it had been necessary to turn up in waiting rooms in a wheelchair several times, bringing my camping bed, eye-mask and ear defenders with me. That made the nurses far more helpful than they have been the times I have forced myself to sit in a chair. They understand that no one brings a camping bed with them unless it is necessary. This has removed the vast majority of my fear of professionals.

It is far less scary being different in public if you have figured out ahead of time what you will say if people ask questions or make comments. People usually ask out of curiosity or consideration. Scepticism often comes from ignorance, not distrust. Giving simple, honest answers without being defensive or aggressive, is what works best. But if someone says something really rude, it is, of course, permissible to answer back.

Good communication can prevent a number of misunderstandings, but does not solve all problems.

Both Stacey and Claire point out that being different can have unexpected consequences. Stacey says:

> *"One thing you have to do when you get ill is forget other people's opinions, not so easy I know but this is your life, one life and your health on this earth so forget them. Plus you might inspire them with challenges in their life; they're not necessarily thinking negative thoughts towards you."*

Claire says:

> *"You get to the stage where it's more important to do what you enjoy than to care what people think... This is hard to get over; but you might come up with a much better way of doing things."*

USING AIDS AND ASSISTANCE

Just as in other invisible illnesses, people with ME are allowed to use aids and ask for assistance. Stacey says:

"You have a 'real' disease and if we all portray this it will get accepted more and ignorance will become more and more diminished. Please get as much assistance as you can, this will be the biggest help, especially emotionally. Don't, obviously, be pushed beyond your limit by them however."

Nikki says:

"Plenty of people with milder conditions use them and I want my life back. It's just a chair with wheels on. Most people use chairs, they also use cars which are large metal boxes with wheels on... I wish I'd done it sooner and been able to do more before I really relapsed and lost those chances to use equipment when it would have opened up more opportunities."

Victoria, too, agrees that it is important to view aids from a positive angle:

"See them as energy-savers and enablers and most people with disabilities can walk a few steps (for example) so you're just as entitled."

IT IS NOT YOUR FAULT

Both experience and research show that the limits people with ME have are still there even when the patients do not push themselves. This shows that ME is not a result of overexertion. Nor is it true that it is the most severely ill who have pushed themselves the furthest. There are examples of patients who push themselves hard, but remain relatively well, while others have become very ill without having pushed themselves hard at all.

The Australian researchers Ian Hickie and Andrew Lloyd followed a group of patients with several types of acute viral infections for several years in order to see which of them got ME afterwards, and which factors were of importance for whether they got ME or not. The greatest risk factor for getting ME was how severe the original viral infection was, while factors such as age and psychological health had no effect.

The British researchers Derek Pheby and Lisa Saffron found that the most important factors for becoming severely ill with ME was lack of support from their doctor, a long wait for a diagnosis and how severe the original infection was. Women were also more liable to get severe ME than men. Perfectionism, on the other hand, had no significance on the development of the illness.

How severe a viral infection you get is something you have no control over. Therefore, there is no basis for saying that ME patients cause their own illness. Nor is there anything in the research that suggests that it is the ME patient's own fault that they are ill, or that they give themselves serious relapses. The health support for ME patients is, unfortunately, still sporadic and often lacking, so that one often does not get correct information and training in pacing. It is absolutely wrong for patients to blame themselves when the lack of support from the health service and society is so extensive. Most understand this with their head, even if they feel as if they are to blame.

Some of the reason for the guilt is that it is a natural part of the grieving process, which Jill Moss points out in her book *Somebody help ME*. Becoming chronically ill involves grief. Even when there is no reason to feel guilty at all, a person who is grieving will usually feel that something is their fault.

MANAGING GUILT

When you are ridden by guilt it helps a lot to talk to others about it. Other people usually find it easier to put things in perspective and remind you that you are not as hopeless as you feel right now. We all have something to be proud of. When you are feeling down it is easier to think about what you are and what you have achieved if you have made a written list. If you, despite this, feel that you need more help to rid yourself of the guilt, you can contact a psychologist. Psychiatrist (and ME patient) Fred Friedberg has a good section on this in his book *Coping with Chronic Fatigue Syndrome: Nine Things You Can Do*. Details of the book are in the reference list.

Nikki says:

> *"At no point have I ever thought pacing making me less ill could mean it's my fault I'm sick! All it proves is that I've taken control of the variables I can influence and that I have the power to get the very best out of the potential my body is capable of. This is the same for many chronic illnesses from cancer, to diabetes or arthritis. I've*

lost enough control as it is. I want to be able to make the most of what I've got left."

OVERACTIVITY CAN GIVE EMOTIONAL INSTABILITY

Overexertion can often cause unstable moods. You may become irritable, giggly and given to laughter, get acute angry outbursts or a tendency towards panic. This also happens to people who are usually harmonious and emotionally stable. Some find they become acutely depressed by overexertion. This occurs perhaps more frequently with cognitive overexertion. If the overexertion continues, the symptoms may continue. When depression or other emotions are caused by overexertion, pacing is a very effective treatment. The symptoms often disappear quickly when you get enough rest, but in people with severe ME it can take longer.

DEPRESSION, GRIEF AND UNSTABLE MOODS

It is important to remember that pacing is not about doing as little as possible for as long as possible. Pacing is about finding out how much activity is just right for your body, and staying within those limits. The problem is that what is right for your body is often too little for your soul.

Sometimes people with ME get clinical depression, that is that they feel as though they are constantly lying at the bottom of a black hole they can't manage to climb out of. Amy points out that it is a good idea to ask for help early on, because ME and depression is not a good combination. She continues:

> *"It's natural to be depressed in our situation. Finding ways to distract ourselves from our situation isn't easy but it's important we do... It's important to recognise that our illness and its limitations can bring clinical depression; depression isn't what made us ill, rather it can be the result of being so incapacitated."*

The healthcare system has several different options. Your doctor can send you to one that is relevant. It can be particularly useful to contact a psychologist with experience of teaching coping skills to patients with chronic illness and disability, because these psychologists will more easily understand that the depression is a result of being chronically ill and not the other way around.

PACING WHEN YOU FEEL LIFE IS TOUGH

Not everyone reacts the same way when they feel down. Some try to distract themselves from sad thoughts, while others become drained of initiative. If you are among those who distract themselves when you are sad, you have to find out how you can avoid overexertion when you are depressed. One trick is to use relaxation CDs, because these both supply distraction and rest at once, but not everyone is well enough for this.

If you belong to the group that loses initiative, it might not be an idea to do less when you are sad, since you can end up doing too little. In addition, this can worsen the feeling of hopelessness, since you have too few pleasant experiences during the day. It might work better to stick to the usual routine. Chapter 6 is about how to make a routine that is suitable on both good and bad days.

TAKING CARE OF YOURSELF EMOTIONALLY

There are events and activities that drain you emotionally and others that recharge your emotional batteries. To have a good quality of life there has to be a balance between the things that drag you down and the things that lift you up. When you feel that there is a lot dragging you down, you can consciously prioritise activities that recharge your emotional batteries. This way you can hinder the depression from getting worse than absolutely necessary and, best case, avoid getting depressed. One way to do it is to make a box full of funny articles and comics, videos, audio books, or the like that can cheer you up on bad days. Amy, who has severe ME, suggests the following:

> "I try to have something good in each day, whether it is something nice to eat or a favourite activity or looking at a pretty picture..."

Stacey, who has moderate ME, mentions:

> "Whenever you can get outside, even just in the garden on a chair and feel well enough to do it, even if you feel like it won't help your mood, do it, it will. Also, try changing things around in your environment for a boost, some new decorations, smells, flowers, here and there. Get someone to do your hair different, etc. I know this won't help everyone."

Dr. Darrel Ho-Yen recommends to his patients to laugh several times every day, since research has shown that this increases the amount of NK-cells (natural killer cells) in your blood.

Stacey says;

> *"Make sure you concentrate on building up a good support group, join an ME charity, they have social groups, all online to help you through this, talk to a professional if you feel it's not improving. But don't see this as weakness or you not coping, you're dealing with a huge amount of isolation and you're human."*

There are a number of books on managing the emotional impact of chronic illness that can be borrowed at the library or bought in a book shop. Be aware that some of these books give advice on diet, exercise and other things that might not be appropriate for people with ME. You have to be prepared to pick out the relevant things. A good English book is *Sick and Tired of Feeling Sick and Tired – Living with Invisible Chronic Illness* by Paul J. Donoghue and Mary E. Siegel. Books on managing the emotional impact are of interest to people who want to learn as much as possible about coping strategies, but do not have emotional problems that need treatment. If you have fairly serious emotional problems you should get professional assistance.

DON'T GIVE UP!

It is tempting to stop pacing if you feel much better. This is a very dangerous idea. If someone with ME lets themselves off the leash and forgets to listen to the body's signals, they will quickly end up with a relapse. Even if you are almost well you can still have serious relapses. It might sound like a straight-jacket to have to continue pacing forever, but it is not really. Learning to recharge your batteries is a useful lesson for everyone, even people who are healthy. Pacing long-term is discussed in Chapter 9, 'Pacing in the Short and Long Term' and in the section on getting better in Chapter 10.

Sarah says:

> *"Pacing is however very personal so do what works for you or it is pointless trying as you will be unable to maintain it long-term...*

Pacing is meant to help so if you don't feel relaxed and comfortable with the way you are doing it then you are doing it wrong! Make it fit into your life then you will soon stop thinking of it as a technique but more as a way of life, and adjust it as your health improves or declines."

REWARD YOURSELF

Since pacing is such a tough management method it is important to give yourself some rewards.

Victoria says:

> *"It's important to give yourself treats every now and then. Plan something fun just beyond your usual boundaries once a month. I find this is important not only emotionally, but a good way to test where you are health-wise."*

Caroline says:

> *"Reward yourself when you have been good at pacing. The reward can be anything just as long as it is something you like. In the choice between the whip and the carrot, choose the carrot."*

It is so important to spend some of your energy on things you love to do that it cannot be underlined enough. This is what makes it possible to stand pacing in the long run. A lot of the desperation disappears when you discover that it is possible to have fun even with ME, just in a different way than before.

YOU ARE NOT THE ILLNESS

> *"Nobody can do everything, not even really healthy people. We all have to make choices. I can still do little things, and while sometimes that doesn't feel like enough I tend to remind myself how much more I can do now and how much I longed to be able to do this much when I was very sick. Once you've been really sick and had almost everything taken away I stopped making so many rules for myself. I can still offer support and friendship to my friends and*

CHAPTER 14: ACCEPTING PACING

family, which is the most important thing. Having friends who understand to share the frustrations with makes it easier to bear them." says Nikki.

Modern society places a great deal of weight on what you do, not who you are. It can be very difficult to free yourself from this and try to see yourself as a real person even if you cannot do as much as everyone else. It can be useful to make a list of the things you appreciate most in the people you are fond of. The list will probably include words like 'loving' and 'warm', 'full of insight' or other words for qualities, not words like 'mows the lawn regularly'. When you have put into words the qualities in others that you appreciate the most, you can ask the people you care about what they appreciate most in you. The answer will most likely not be that you do the dishes every day. So it is not true that you are worthless just because you cannot do everything you did before.

As Amy says:

> *"ME may rule our lives but we don't have to be defined by it; I am more than ME, I am me."*

****

Pacing can be a challenge emotionally. It is important not to hide feelings away and pretend they are not there, but instead to look openly and honestly at the problems. There is often something that can be done, either by thinking differently or by figuring out practical solutions that make pacing easier. When there are many challenges it can help to think that it is easier to keep going with a management strategy that works, than to have a rough time because you are not pacing activities. It is like Stacey says: *"It is a grind day in and day out but you'll be forever proud of your resilience."*

TASKS

1 Which thoughts and feelings in this chapter did you recognise?

2 Think through whether you have experienced other thoughts and feelings than those described in this chapter. Put into words which aspects of pacing you find most difficult right now. If you think it is hard to describe them in words, you can try to draw, paint or choose music that you feel represents the situation.

DONNA HOPKINS, 48 YEARS OF AGE

"I think it is called motivation. I've had ME for 20 years, and consider myself motivated, but still have difficulties with sometimes thinking some of the thoughts mentioned in the previous chapter. I think the answer may lie in Buddhist type thought e.g. 'it is what is' i.e. if you accept your current situation, then you change your patterns of thinking to more positive. Then you take an event such as your birthday when you have felt all the love and affection from people, so you are on a 'high' then, like me, you say I don't like my situation right now, and I feel angry that I'm in it. Then you write down in a book all your anger. This could take weeks. You could also talk to a counsellor. So anger's gone. You are left more at peace, and then you say there are things suggested I could do to get better. I could chose to ignore this advice or if I want I could chose to try the pacing. No one else is forcing me. It's my choice. And say, I with this illness am in a new situation, the old thought patterns and ways of doing stuff don't apply now. I am me, and I am special, and doing half an activity is good now because it suits me at this time in my life. I am willing to try this and let go of past thoughts and expectations. In time I will be able to do the full activity but now is now, and now a different approach is needed. One person said to me they got better after they said to themselves, "I no longer fight this illness, ME. I accept I have ME, I am not angry."

SUMMARY OF CHAPTER 15

1. An activity diary can be interpreted on three levels:

   • the micro level is about the individual activity.

   • the intermediate level is about individual days.

   • the macro level is about studying longer periods.

2. To interpret the diary on micro and intermediate level you need a detailed diary. The best thing is to look at bad, average and good days, but if you cannot manage to keep the diary for several days, you can make do with one bad day.

3. When interpreting on the micro level the goal is to find out how long you can do a given activity without getting tired or without the symptoms changing. Activities that lead to changes in symptoms must be done for a shorter time and/or more gently, with the help of energy conservation techniques.

4. When interpreting on the intermediate level the goal is to find out how to spread activities during the day in such a way that you can keep up your strength and recharge your batteries.

5. At the intermediate level you look at the balance between activity and rest, between physical, mental and social activities, and at ups and downs in your condition throughout the day.

CHAPTER 15:

LEARN TO INTERPRET THE ACTIVITY DIARY

INTRODUCTION

When you have kept a diary for a bit you are ready to learn how to analyse and interpret it in order to find out which activity level is right for you. The diary can be interpreted at three levels, micro, intermediate, and macro. Pacing at the micro level is all about pacing individual activities. At the intermediate level it is about pacing the activities during a whole day, while the macro level is all about pacing over longer periods of time, like from day to day, week to week or month to month. In this chapter the focus is on interpreting the diary on the micro and intermediate levels. For this you need a detailed diary for preferably a few days. Interpreting the activity diary at the macro level is discussed in the next chapter.

MICRO-LEVEL INTERPRETATION

Micro-level interpretation has three purposes.

- Evaluating the symptom level
  Learn to evaluate the symptom level and which activity level is realistic.

- Recognising the warning signs
  Learn to recognise warning signs which show that you are doing too much.

- Finding the right length of activities
  Find out how long you can do an activity without getting warning signs.

To learn all this you have to ask the right questions about the facts recorded in the diary. It is useful to ask the following questions:

BEFORE THE ACTIVITY:

How high was the symptom level and which symptoms did you have? Was the activity a realistic and sensible choice based on this?

DURING THE ACTIVITY:

Did you get any symptoms while doing the activity? How long did it take before you got the symptoms? Include warning signs that are so small that you perhaps don't think of them as symptoms, i.e. a woolly feeling that it might be time to stop.

AFTER THE ACTIVITY:

How did you feel after the activity? If you got symptom increases, how long did it take to rest them away?

JOHN

Figures 1, 2 and 3 show three excerpts from John's diary; he has moderate ME. In Figure 1 John has a high symptom level: 7 out of 10. He chooses to go for an hour's shopping trip anyway. During the trip he gets a number of symptoms: pain, dizziness and exhaustion. Afterwards he is so exhausted that he falls asleep on the sofa for three hours. The rest of the day he is totally worn out and the day after he feels worse than usual. It is very clear here that John would have benefited by choosing a less tiring activity.

FIGURE 1 – JOHN'S DIARY

EXAMPLE A:

SYMPTOM LEVEL FROM 0-10 BEFORE THE ACTIVITY	TYPE OF ACTIVITY OR REST	TIME	SYMPTOMS	SYMPTOM LEVEL FROM 0-10 AFTER THE ACTIVITY
7	Shopping trip	1 h	Pain, dizziness, worn out	10
10	Slept on the sofa	3 h	Exhausted	9

Both the high symptom level at the beginning, the increasing symptoms along the way, and the strong reaction afterwards, show this. If John had run out of food and therefore had to go shopping, he could have cut down the time to 15 minutes. Then he would probably have felt quite tired for a while afterwards, but probably not have had the rest of the day spoiled.

In Figure 2 John does not feel too bad before the activity. The symptom level is 4 out of 10 possible. He chooses to write an email for 20 minutes. After 11 minutes he begins to feel that it is time to stop. After 12 minutes his hands get tired. A minute later he gets pain in his hands and after 18 minutes he begins to get tired in his whole body and gets concentration problems. Afterwards he feels worse for a while.

FIGURE 2 — JOHN'S DIARY

EXAMPLE B:

SYMPTOM LEVEL FROM 0-10 BEFORE THE ACTIVITY	TYPE OF ACTIVITY OR REST	TIME	SYMPTOMS	SYMPTOM LEVEL FROM 0-10 AFTER THE ACTIVITY
4	Wrote email	20 min.	After 11 min: woolly feeling of it being time to stop After 12 min: Hands tired After 13 min: Pain in hands After 18 min: Tired in whole body, concentration problems	7
7	Rest	40 min.	Exhausted	5

The symptom level was evaluated as 7 out of 10, but after a good rest break he felt better again. Here it looks as if John has chosen a realistic activity for his symptom level. But he keeps going for a little too long. He overlooks the first warning sign, namely the vague feeling that it is time to stop, and goes on until his whole body is tired. That is why he needs to spend time recovering again afterwards. If John had stopped after 10 minutes, that is before he got any symptom increase at all, the whole rest break would have been healing rest. Then he would probably also only have needed a shorter rest.

In Figure 3 John has a bad day. The symptom level is 8 out of 10 because he has pain both in his eyes and legs. John chooses to listen to an audio book for 10 minutes. There are no warning signs while he is doing it, and after the rest break he actually feels a bit better – 7 out of 10. John has clearly chosen a sensible activity on the basis of the symptoms he has. He chooses an activity that has nothing to do with the painful body parts. Also, John stops so early that he doesn't get worse, and actually feels better after the rest break. Figure 3 is an ideal example. It is, of course, not always possible to stop early enough and rest long enough to feel better afterwards, but it is amazing how much it helps to try.

FIGURE 3 – JOHN'S DIARY

EXAMPLE C:

SYMPTOM LEVEL FROM 0-10 BEFORE THE ACTIVITY:	TYPE OF ACTIVITY OR REST:	TIME:	SYMPTOMS:	SYMPTOM LEVEL FROM 0-10 AFTER THE ACTIVITY
8	Audio book	10 min.	No symptoms occur	8
8	Rest	30 min.	Improvement	7

Pacing at the micro level is one of the most important things people with ME can learn. Once you have mastered this you have learned an important tool for keeping the illness in check. When you have learned pacing at the micro level it is not difficult to do it at the intermediate and macro levels too. On the other hand it is almost impossible to manage pacing at the intermediate and macro levels if you don't understand or master the micro level. You should focus on the micro level to begin with.

INTERPRETING AT THE INTERMEDIATE LEVEL

Pacing at the intermediate level is a bit more complicated than at the micro level. Just as in the micro level each separate activity is kept within what you can tolerate. In addition, the total amount of activity must be kept within the limits you have. This means that there are more questions to ask and more details to keep an eye on. The more you know about what your body can take of the separate activities, the easier it is to evaluate how much you can take in a day. First we look at the questions to ask, and then we discuss how to use the information.

When you are going to interpret a whole day from the activity diary, you can use the following questions:

- Planning:

  Were the planned activities and the length of them realistic? (Could the activities be done without getting a worsening of symptoms during the day, nor in the days afterwards?)

- Symptoms:

  How did the symptoms develop during the day? Were there peaks and troughs, steady improvement or steady deterioration? How did the symptoms develop over the following days? Did you get a delayed symptom flare? How did the symptoms develop during each separate activity, and during possible rest breaks?

- Activities:

  Were the activity spells spread evenly during the day? Was there a difference in the lengths? Were there different types of activity (physical, mental and social, both fun and work-like, and activities that use different body parts)?

- Rest:

  Did you take rest breaks and were they long enough? Were these used to get over activities that had tired you, or did you rest even though you felt ok?

- Afterwards:

  Was this an activity level that you could use every day, or was it so tiring that the symptoms got worse, either at the end of the day, next day, or in the following days? I discuss this in greater detail later in the chapter.

Realistic planning has to do with planning a number of activities that you can accomplish without getting worse. This will often mean that you must choose one thing or the other, but not both. A moderately ill person could perhaps shop for a birthday gift or go the birthday party, but not do both on the same day. A person who is too ill to go out, might manage a short visit or a short phone call, but not both. Occasionally, you may find that you are forced, or very much wish, to plan activities that make you worse over the following day or days. Then it is important to remember two things. First, the pleasure or usefulness you get from the activity must stand in a reasonable relation to the discomfort you get from the relapse, so that you feel that it was worth the effort. Secondly, it is important that this sort of peak is so unusual that it does not eat up any surplus you have built up or hinder any improvement you may be experiencing.

When it comes to symptom flares during the day, it is important to find out whether these are caused by the activity level, or by other causes. Very often symptom flares are due to having done too much. It might be that a single activity was kept up for too long, or that the total amount of small activity periods became too much. This latter situation often leads to feeling worse and worse during the day or that there are periods during the day when you can manage to do more and others when you cannot manage anything. In order to improve as quickly as possible it is very important to make sure you keep a good safety margin throughout the day. Activity periods that lead to symptom flares should therefore be kept so short that they do not change the symptom level. It can often help to vary between different types of activities by, for example, not using the same body part all the time. Other times you need more and longer rest breaks.

Be aware that people with ME often have a time of day when they feel worse. Examples of reasons for this could be that you wake up dehydrated and have to drink enough to feel more or less ok, or that you get worn out by digesting meals. Often people are worse in the morning and feel better in the afternoon and evening, but it can also be the other way around. It is important to take into consideration these kinds of fluctuations during the day. You should do less in the bad periods to avoid making them worse, but also try to make sure that you do not do too much during the good periods. That way you can avoid making the bad periods worse than they have to be. One of the most common reasons for fluctuations during the course of the day is that periods of overactivity are followed by symptom flares. If that is the case, then you are worse in the morning because you did too much the evening before, or worse in the evening because you did too much in the morning. This type of peak and trough can be prevented with pacing. Fluctuations that are caused by other things do not always get better by pacing yourself. They may have to be handled differently.

IDA — GREATER VARIATION

Figure 4 shows an excerpt from Ida's activity diary. Ida has moderate ME, but just as with the other examples in this chapter, the principles apply to any ability level.

FIGURE 4 — IDA'S DIARY

SYMPTOM LEVEL FROM 0-10 BEFORE ACTIVITY	TYPE OF ACTIVITY	TIME OF DAY	TIME	SYMPTOMS	SYMPTOM LEVEL FROM 0-10 AFTER ACTIVITY
6	Made lunch	2pm – 2.05pm	5 min.	No symptom change	6
6	Watched DVD and ate lunch on sofa	2.05pm – 3.30pm	85 min.	Head tired from DVD	7
7	Phone call	3.30pm – 4.30pm	60 min.	Wired, hard to stop talking	8
8	Watch TV	4.30pm – 6.00pm	90 min.	Gradually more concentration problems, more and more exhausted, pain	9
9	Fell asleep on sofa	6.00pm – 6.30pm	30 min.		8

The most striking thing about Ida's diary is that all activities are mental, except making lunch. Also, the activity periods are long and not very varied, and there are no rest breaks. Ida's symptoms get worse and worse and it ends with her falling asleep on the sofa. If Ida had chosen shorter spells and greater variation between activities, she may well have been able to avoid the symptom flaring that comes in the afternoon. She could also have planned a rest break during the afternoon instead of waiting until she was so exhausted that she fell asleep. Her day could have looked like the one in Figure 5.

FIGURE 5 — IDA'S REVISED DIARY

SYMPTOM LEVEL FROM 0-10 BEFORE ACTIVITY	TYPE OF ACTIVITY	TIME OF DAY	TIME	SYMPTOMS	SYMPTOM LEVEL FROM 0-10 AFTER ACTIVITY
6	Making lunch	2.00pm – 2.05pm	5 min.	Unchanged symptoms	6
6	Eating lunch	2.05pm – 2.15pm	10 min.	-:-	6
6	DVD	2.15pm – 2.40pm	25 min.	-:-	6
6	Washing dishes while sitting down	2.40pm – 3.00pm	20 min.	-:-	6
6	Rest	3.00pm – 3.10pm	10 min.	-:-	6
6	DVD	3.10pm – 3.35pm	25 min.	-:-	6
6	Walk	3.35pm – 3.45pm	10 min.	-:-	6
6	Rest	3.45pm – 4.05pm	20 min.	A bit better	5

Chapter 10 discusses healing rest and repairing rest. Since it looks like healing rest often leads to improvement, it is important to study the activity diary to see if you get healing rest during the day. In Figure 4 Ida does not rest until she is exhausted. This is a classic example of repairing rest. This kind of rest means that you get over the overexertions, but your condition is less likely to improve. In Figure 5 Ida takes short, frequent rest breaks to avoid getting worn out during the day. After her walk she takes an extra-long rest. That way she gets healing rest and actually feels better during the day. Ida feels that it is too big a change for her body to go directly from a rest to a physical activity like walking. Others prefer to rest just before a more demanding activity. This is an area where you must experiment cautiously to find out what works best for you.

FIGURE 6 – MARTIN'S ACTIVITY DIARY

SYMPTOM LEVEL FROM 0-10 BEFORE ACTIVITY	TIME OF DAY	TIME	TYPE OF ACTIVITY	SYMPTOMS	SYMPTOM LEVEL FROM 0-10 AFTER ACTIVITY	SYMPTOM LEVEL FROM 0-10 BEFORE ACTIVITY
4	8.45am – 9.45am	1h	Morning routine: Wash, dress, breakfast, etc.	Not demanding	No change	4
4	9.45am – 10.00am	15 min.	Taxi to school	Not demanding	-:-	4
4	10.00am – 10.10am	10 min.	Met friends	Main activity	-:-	4
4	10.10am – 11.40am	1h 30 min	School	Main activity	Head and body gradually more tired	4
5	11.40am – 12.20pm	40 min.	Went to store for lunch with friends	Main activity	Legs tired, dizzy from standing in line	5
5	12.20pm – 1.50pm	1h 30 min.	School	Main activity	Head and body gradually more tired	7
6	1.50 pm – 2.00pm	10 min.	Talked to friends	Main activity	No change	7
7	2.00pm – 2.15pm	15 min.	Taxi home	Not demanding	-:-	7
7	2.15pm – 2.30pm	15 min.	Made sandwich and ate it	Not demanding	-:-	7
7	2.30pm – 3.30pm	1h	Watched TV	Not demanding	Gradually less tired	5
5	3.30pm – 4.30pm	1h	Played computer games	Main activity	Headache + concentration problems towards the end	7
7	4.30pm – 5.30pm	1h	Watched dinner being made and talked to parents	Not demanding	No change	7
7	5.30pm – 6.00pm	30 min.	Ate dinner	Not demanding	Gradually clearer head	6
6	6.00pm – 7.00pm	1h	Homework	Main activity	Head tired	8
8	7.00pm – 7.30pm	30 min.	Cleaned hamster cage and played with hamster	Not demanding	Head gradually better	7
7	7.30pm – 7.45pm	15 min.	Walk	Main activity	Legs a bit tired	7
7	7.45pm – 9.45pm	2h	Watched TV	Not demanding	Legs quickly better, head gradually worse	8
8	9.45pm – 10.00pm	15 min.	Evening routine: Brush teeth, undress	Not demanding	No change	8
8	10.00pm		Bedtime		Head tired, hard to sleep, overstimulated	8

MARTIN — VARIATION IN INTENSITY

Like Ida, Martin is not bedbound either and has become a bit better. Martin's activity diary is shown in Figure 6. He can manage four hours at school each day and can spend time with friends at weekends. Martin can get through the day without breaks, but gets quite tired. On Martin's level it is important to distinguish between main activities (demanding) and less demanding activities. You can read about these two types in Chapter 5. By switching between main activities and less demanding activities during the day you can avoid draining your energy. It is especially important to make sure that the demanding activity periods are not too long.

When you manage to get through the day without rest breaks, it can be very helpful to put in a rest break of five minutes every hour. This is done in Martin's revised diary which is shown in Figure 7. In addition he adds a long relaxation period right after coming home from school in order to charge his batteries again as quickly as possible. In the revised diary he also shortens his main activities and splits them up so that he avoids peaks and troughs in his energy level.

FIGURE 7 — MARTIN'S REVISED ACTIVITY DIARY

SYMPTOM LEVEL FROM 0-10 BEFORE THE ACTIVITY	TIME OF DAY	TIME	TYPE OF ACTIVITY	INTENSITY	SYMPTOMS	SYMPTOM LEVEL FROM 0-10 AFTER THE ACTIVITY
4	8.45am–9.45am	1 h	Morning routine: Wash, dress	Not demanding	No change	4
4	9.45am–10.00am	15 min.	Taxi to school	Not demanding	-:-	4
4	10.00am–10.10am	10 min.	Meet friends	Main activity	-:-	4
4	10.10am–11.40am	1h 30 min.	School	Main activity	-:-	4
4	11.40am–12.00pm	20 min.	Rest	Rest	-:-	4
4	12.00pm–12.20pm	20 min.	Meet friends at lunch	Main activity	-:-	4
4	12.20pm–1.50 pm	1h 30 min.	School	Main activity	Body and head gradually more tired	5

5	1.50pm – 2.00pm	10 min.	Rest	Rest	No change	5
5	2.00pm – 2.15pm	15 min.	Taxi home	Not demanding	-:-	5
5	2.15pm – 2.30pm	15 min.	Made sandwich and ate	Not demanding	-:-	5
5	2.30pm – 3.00pm	30 min.	Relaxation exercises	Rest	Better generally	3
3	3.00pm – 3.55pm	1h55 min	Watched TV	Not demanding	No change	3
3	3.55pm – 4.00pm	5 min.	Rest	Rest	-:-	3
3	4.00pm– 4.30pm	30 min.	Homework	Main activity	-:-	3
3	4.30pm – 5.00pm	30 min.	Watch dinner be made. Talked to parents.	Not demanding	-:-	3
3	5.00pm – 5.05pm	5 min.	Rest	Rest	-:-	3
3	5.05pm – 5.30pm	25 min.	Watch dinner be made. Talked to parents.	Not demanding	-:-	3
3	5.30pm – 5.55pm	25 min.	Ate dinner	Not demanding	-:-	3
3	5.55pm – 6.00pm	5 min.	Rest	Rest	-:-	3
3	6.00pm – 6.30pm	30 min.	Homework	Main activity	Head a bit more tired	4
4	6.30pm – 7.00pm	30 min.	Cleaned hamster cage and played with hamster	Not demanding	Head better	3
3	7.00pm – 7.05pm	5 min.	Rest	Rest	No change	3
3	7.05pm – 7.30pm	25 min.	Played computer games	Main activity	Head a bit more tired	4
4	7.30pm – 8.00pm	30 min.	Watched TV	Not demanding	No change	4
4	8.00pm – 8.05pm	5 min.	Rest during commercial break	Rest	-:-	4
4	8.05pm – 8.30pm	25 min.	Watched TV	Not demanding	-:-	4
4	8.30pm – 8.45pm	15 min.	Walk	Main activity	-:-	4
4	8.45pm – 9.45pm	1 h	Warm caffeine-free drink. Listened to music to relax.	Not demanding	Better generally	3
3	9.45pm – 10.00pm	15 min.	Evening routine: brush teeth, undress	Not demanding	No change	3
3	10.00pm		Bedtime			

PETER — SHORTER ACTIVITY PERIODS

One of the patterns you should be on the guard against is long activity periods that need disproportionately long rest breaks afterwards. In Figure 8 there is an extract from Peter's diary. Peter has severe ME and spends his days in bed. On this day he is spending a little time on his computer, but gets over-eager and goes on for half an hour. Then he is so exhausted that he has to rest for two hours afterwards. The next two activity periods are only 5 minutes long each, which leads to little or no symptom increase. It is easy to see that 30 minutes are too much for Peter, while five minutes seems to be about right.

FIGURE 8 — PETER'S ACTIVITY DIARY

SYMPTOM LEVEL FROM 0-10 BEFORE THE ACTIVITY	TIME OF DAY	TIME	TYPE OF ACTIVITY	INTENSITY	SYMPTOMS	SYMPTOM LEVEL FROM 0-10 AFTER THE ACTIVITY
7	11.30am – 12.00pm	30 min.	Computer in bed	Main activity	Headache, pain in eyes and arms, concentration problems, very tired	9
9	12.00pm – 2.00pm	2h	Rest	Rest	Slowly better	7
7	2.00pm – 2.05pm	5 min.	Ate sandwich in bed	Main activity	Arm and jaw a bit sore	8
8	2.05pm – 2.35pm	30 min.	Rest	Rest	Better again	7
7	2.35pm – 2.40pm	5 min.	Audio book	Not demanding	No symptom increase	7

Next day Peter plans his day as shown in Figure 9. Here, all activity periods are five minutes long. He still has to rest a lot, but he avoids a very boring two hour rest after the overexertion. Also, Peter makes sure to switch between different types of activity, so that he does not use the same body part or body function all the time. The spells of five minutes are only examples. In practice, Peter can do some activities for eight minutes and others for only two minutes.

FIGURE 9 — PETER'S REVISED ACTIVITY DIARY

SYMPTOM LEVEL FROM 0-10 BEFORE ACTIVITY	TIME OF DAY	TIME	TYPE OF ACTIVITY	INTENSITY	STRAINED AREA	SYMPTOM LEVEL FROM 0-10 AFTER ACTIVITY
7	11.00am-11.05am	5 min.	Computer	Main activity	Mental, eyes, arms	7
7	11.05am – 11.35am	30 min.	Rest	Rest		7
7	11.35am – 11.40am	5 min.	Toilet	Main activity	Physical, legs	7
7	11.40am – 12.10pm	30 min.	Rest	Rest		7
7	12.10pm – 12.15pm	5 min.	Puzzle	Not demanding	Mental, eyes, arms	7
7	12.15pm – 12.45pm	30 min.	Rest	Rest		7
7	12.45pm – 12.50pm	5 min.	Audio book	Not demanding	Mental, ears	7
7	12.50pm – 1.20pm	30 min.	Rest	Rest		7
7	1.20pm – 1.25pm	5 min.	Sandwich	Main activity	Physical, arms, jaw	7
7	1.25pm – 1.55pm	30 min.	Rest	Rest		7
7	1.55pm – 2.00pm	5 min.	Computer again	Main activity	Mental, eyes, arms	7

LENA — SHORT AND LONG REST BREAKS

Lena is also bedbound, but is considerably sicker than Peter. She needs assistance with everything, and cannot lift herself over on to the bedpan. A challenge Lena has is that she needs long rest breaks between each activity, but at the same time she needs frequent meals. Since there are only 24 hours in a day she has found a compromise by having some short and some longer rest breaks. This works well for her. An excerpt from Lena's diary is shown in Figure 10. The conversation at the end of the example got to be far too long. With a conversation of only a minute Lena would be able to avoid the big symptom flare. On Lena's level people commonly need to convey messages over several days, and split meals and personal hygiene into small sessions, etc. That makes it very important to have people around you who are very disciplined.

FIGURE 10 – LENA'S ACTIVITY DIARY

SYMPTOM LEVEL FROM 0-10 BEFORE ACTIVITY	TIME OF DAY	TIME	TYPE OF ACTIVITY	INTENSITY	SYMPTOMS	STRAINED AREA	SYMPTOM LEVEL FROM 0-10 AFTER ACTIVITY
9	9.00am – 9.02am	2 min.	Teeth brushing done by assistant while Lena lies flat	Not demanding		Physical, mouth	9
9	9.02am – 9.32am	30 min.	Rest				9
9	9.32am – 9.37am	5 min.	Fed porridge for breakfast	Main activity		Physical, mouth and stomach	9
9	9.37am – 9.42am	5 min.	Rest				9
9	9.42am – 9.47am	5 min.	More breakfast	Main activity	Mouth pain, tired from digesting	Physical, mouth and stomach	9.5
9.5	9.47am – 10.47am	1 h	Rest				9
9	10.47am – 10.50am	3 min.	Bed pan, plus change of position to prevent pressure sores	Main activity		Physical	9
9	10.50am – 11.50am	1 h	Rest				9
9		10 sec.	Look at picture	Not demanding		Mental, eyes	9
9	11.50am – 12.05pm	15 min.	Rest				9
9	12.05pm – 12.10pm	5 min.	Lunch, drink smoothie with straw	Main activity		Physical, mouth and stomach	9
9	12.10pm – 12.15pm	5 min.	Rest				9
9	12.15pm – 12.20pm	5 min.	Lunch continued	Main activity	Pain in mouth, tired from digesting	Physical, mouth and stomach	9.5
9.5	12.20pm – 12.50pm	30 min.	Rest				9
9	12.50pm – 12.55pm	5 min.	Conversation	Main activity	Exhausted, not able to talk for the next 2 days	Mental	10

HANNA

Hanna is much better and now has mild ME. She has chosen to work 60 per cent so as to have some energy left over to be with her husband and children. When Hanna started working again she worked eight hours, three days a week. Then she was tired when she got home and had to use her days off to recuperate. Now she has a set up where she works six hours, four days a week. That way she still has some energy left over for the family when she gets home from work. After the change, Hanna's diary looks like Figure 11. Hanna's weekly routine can be found in Chapter 5. On the surface, Hanna's life seems quite normal. But she lives more quietly than healthy people. She uses energy conservation techniques and drives a car in situations where others would walk. Hanna manages to practise qigong since the classes are specially designed for people with ME, but more fatiguing things like aerobics would give her a strong symptom increase. Hanna has to be careful to avoid several busy days in a row.

Like Martin, Hanna takes several short rest breaks during the course of the day. She also has a relaxation session after work and a spell lasting ten minutes at lunch. For Hanna this is enough to charge her batteries over the course of the day, as long as she does not do too much. Hanna feels that she gets more out of her day when she structures it. At the same time, her body can now tolerate priority changes at short notice, if she must. That was much more difficult when she was more ill.

FIGURE 11 – HANNA'S ACTIVITY DIARY

SYMPTOM LEVEL FROM 0-10 BEFORE ACTIVITY	TIME OF DAY	TIME	TYPE OF ACTIVITY	INTENSITY	SYMPTOMS	STRAINED AREA	SYMPTOM LEVEL FROM 0-10 AFTER ACTIVITY
2	7.00am – 8.00am	1h	Get up, wash, dress, breakfast with family	Not demanding		Physical, social	2
2	8.00am – 8.40am	40 min.	Drive kids to nursery school	Demanding		Mental, physical	2
2	8.40am– 9.00am	20 min.	Drive to work	Demanding		Mental, physical	2
2	9.00am – 12.00pm	3h	Work	Demanding		Mental, social	2

2	12.00pm – 12.10pm	10 min.	10 min relaxation exercises at lunch. Some two min breathing breaks during workday	Rest			2
2	12.10pm – 3.00pm	2h 50 min	Work	Demanding		Mental, social	3
3	3.00pm – 3.20pm	20 min.	Drive home	Demanding	Tired and concentration problems	Mental, physical	3
3	3.20pm – 3.35pm	15 min.	Relaxation exercises	Rest	Better again		2
2	3.35pm – 3.55pm	30 min.	Knitting	Not demanding		Light physical	2
2	3.55pm – 4.35pm	30 min.	TV	Not demanding		Mental	2
2	4.35pm		Family comes home	Not demanding		Social	2
2	4.35pm – 6.00pm	1h 25 min	Family makes and eats dinner together	Demanding		Social, physical	2
2	6.00pm – 6.10pm	10 min.	Rest 10 mins while kids watch TV	Rest			2
2	6.10pm – 6.30pm	20 min.	Tidy kitchen	Not demanding		Physical	2
2	6.30pm – 7.30pm	1h	Play game with kids	Not demanding		Social	2
2	7.30pm – 8.00pm	30 min.	Read to kids after husband puts them to bed	Not demanding		Mental	2
2	8.00pm – 8.05pm	5 min.	Rest	Rest			2
2	8.05pm – 8.35pm	30 min.	Talk with husband	Not demanding		Social	2
2	8.35pm – 8.50pm	15 min.	Knitting	Not demanding		Physical	2
2	8.50pm – 9.20pm	30 min.	Phone call	Not demanding		Social, mental	2
2	9.20pm – 9.50pm	30 min.	Read book	Not demanding		Mental	2
2	9.50pm – 10.00pm	10 min.	Conversation with husband	Not demanding		Social	2
2	10.00pm – 10.15pm	15 min.	Evening routine	Not demanding		Physical	2

MACRO LEVEL PACING

The last question that must be asked when you interpret the activity diary is how the symptoms and activity level develop over the days that follow. What you have to be aware of here is that it is possible to do too much of one thing, even though the activity level as a whole was not too high. For example, you might have used your arms too much but not the rest of your body. This sort of overexertion should be avoided because it can slow down the healing process in the long run. The same goes for overexertion where you do too much in general and must pay the price for several days afterwards. That sort of pattern has to do with macro level pacing. This will be discussed in the next chapter.

****

Learning to interpret the activity diary makes the diary more than just a monitoring tool. It becomes a tool for understanding your own limits. You start on the micro level and then move on to the next level as you get a good grasp of the tool. After a while you will have collected all the information you need to pace your activities so that they are spread more evenly throughout the day.

TASKS

1 Practise interpreting the diary on the micro level by using the questions in this chapter. Consider which changes you feel could be helpful to you.

2 Make the changes. If they seem overwhelming, take one at a time and give yourself some sort of reward when you manage it.

3 Do not start on the intermediate level until you have a good grasp of the micro level. That way the job of interpreting on the intermediate level is much simpler, and the number of changes on the intermediate level will be far fewer.

4 Make changes on the intermediate level. These can also be done in small chunks.

Interpreting on the macro level is the last stage. Do not start on it until you have read the next chapter.

SUMMARY OF CHAPTER 16

1. Interpreting the activity diary on the macro level is all about looking at how the activity level and the symptom level develop over a longer period.

2. You can make a graph that shows both the activity level and the symptom level. This is easiest if you use a simple diary.

3. You can interpret the graph in order to improve your insight into your own activity patterns.

4. You can, among other things, gain insight into:
   - Which activity level worsens symptoms.
   - Which activity level improves symptoms.
   - Whether there are patterns that repeat themselves.
   - Which stage you are at (for a more detailed description, see Chapter 11).

5. You can make a strategy for pacing based on what you have found out from the graph.

6. Graphs are good for following up long-term and for documenting that the management and treatment strategies you use are effective.

CHAPTER 16:

MACRO LEVEL INTERPRETATION

INTRODUCTION

Pacing on the macro level is about balancing activities from day to day, week to week, and month to month. The principles for pacing at the macro level are the same as those at the micro level. Every day and every period of the day must be kept within the limits of what you experience as comfortable. The difference is that it can be difficult to interpret a normal activity diary when you look at pacing on the macro level. This is because the number of days is so large that you can lose the general view.

There is in other words a need for a simple and surveyable way of showing changes in activity level from day to day over a longer period. The easiest way to do this is to draw a graph. If you use a simple activity diary, it is very simple to make a graph of the numbers from the diary. If you write a detailed diary, drawing a graph is more complicated. There is a system that makes it possible to change the text in the diary to numbers that can be put into the graph. This is explained in Worksheet 8. Because the system involves some arithmetic, many people will need assistance. That is why the simple diary is more suitable for long-term follow-up. You do not need to read Worksheet 8 if you are not going to make a graph from a detailed diary.

MAKING A GRAPH

When you have kept the diary for some days you can draw a graph. You can either use Worksheet 5 (graph sheet for a simple diary), or Worksheet 9 (graph sheet for a detailed diary). You will find both of these at the back of the book. You can also make a graph on any graph paper or squared paper. The graph itself is drawn by marking a point for the number for the activity level and a point for the number for the symptom level for each day. When you have put in the points for the next day, you can draw a line between the points for activity and between the points for symptoms. After a few days you will have two lines, and you can see if there is a connection between the activity level and the symptom level. An example of this sort of connection is that the symptom level goes up if you do more than usual. The purpose of the graph is to see how the activity level develops from day to day and week to week.

The graph has two functions, an analysis function and a monitoring function. By analysing the graph you can see if the activity level follows a certain pattern. That way you get the possibility of changing unfortunate patterns in a better direction. You might possibly discover that things are going well and that you do not need to make any changes. In that case you do not have to worry about whether you are pacing your activities well enough. In order to analyse the graph you need at least two weeks of diary records, sometimes considerably more.

The graph's other function is to record the development of your illness. If your health is deteriorating, the graph might show that your pacing efforts are gradually making the deterioration slow down, or that you are beginning to stabilise. It may also show that certain events, such as strenuous physiotherapy, are causing a stepwise deterioration. This could document which approaches work and which do not work. Even if your health is improving quickly, it seldom moves so fast that you can tell the difference from day to day. It is easier to avoid getting desperate if you have a graph that shows that things are improving. Similarly, it is easier to stick with the pacing when you see that your efforts are gradually bringing you in the right direction, even if you are still in the process of learning the technique.

If you can show that your health is becoming more stable or improving, using the graph, this can reduce some of the pressure that people with ME are often exposed to. For example, you could use it to show health care professionals that pacing is an appropriate strategy.

INTERPRETING THE GRAPH

When interpreting the graph, you can use questions in the same way you did on the micro and intermediate levels:

- Which activity level causes a worsening of symptoms?
- Which activity level leads to an improvement of symptoms?

- Are there patterns that repeat themselves?

- If you have read Chapter 11, which stage are you at?

Graphs from the activity diary often form typical patterns. Some of these patterns can be used as warning signs, while others are favourable. Below you will find an overview of the most important ones, and tips on how to turn unfortunate patterns in a better direction. Most of the graphs are based on actual diaries, but some have been constructed so as to make the patterns show up more clearly.

OVERVIEW OF UNFORTUNATE PATTERNS

Some patterns can be considered as warning signs. Below you will find an overview of the most important patterns.

UNSTABLE ACTIVITY LEVEL

Figure 1 shows an unstable activity level. It is characterised by a big difference between good and bad days. This pattern usually emerges through resting for some days, feeling a little better and then doing far too much. Then you get some bad days and have to rest again. This kind of pattern can be called a rollercoaster pattern. Overactivity quickly leads to worsening of symptoms.

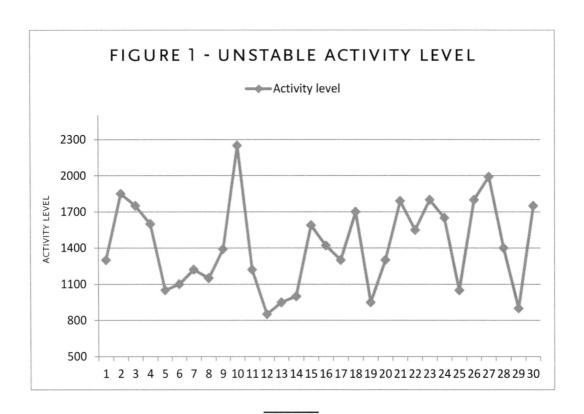

FIGURE 1 - UNSTABLE ACTIVITY LEVEL

ROLLERCOASTER PATTERN

In Figure 2 the rollercoaster pattern is even clearer. Here you can see that the person does not feel too bad on Monday. Therefore, they do a lot on Monday and Tuesday, and this leads to a worsening of their symptoms. During the week the rest leads to symptoms improving again, and the week after this pattern repeats itself. Sometimes this pattern can be seen over much longer time periods. For example, you can do a lot for several weeks, and then crash for several weeks, or for that matter do a lot for several months and then crash for several months. This pattern can also be found on the micro level in the course of a day. Everyone with ME has experienced that a too high activity level during one period of the day leads to a crash landing on the sofa for a while, before you are capable of doing something again. A third type of rollercoaster pattern is having to spend a few days in bed because you have done too much on the other days.

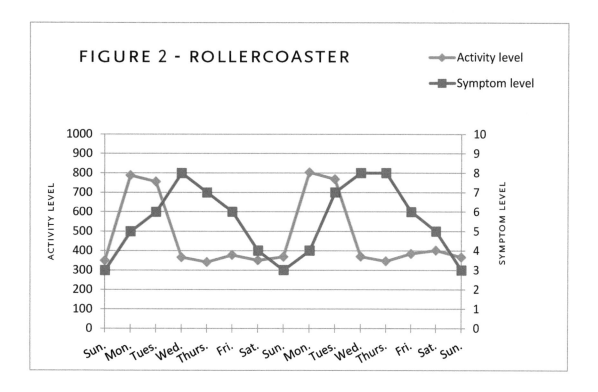

Living with an unstable activity and symptom level is frustrating because you never know how you are going to feel in a few days' time. Therefore, it is almost impossible to plan things. It is also difficult to spot when your condition is improving or getting worse. Unstable improvement is possible, but you never know how long the situation is going to last. This is what characterises the unstable phase. The important thing is to gain stability and improvement. Stability is important because it creates the opportunity to plan and that is something that gives you more power over your own life. Why you want improvement of your condition is not something that needs an explanation. Chapter 11 describes techniques to help stabilise a fluctuating pattern.

HIGH SYMPTOM LEVEL

A high symptom level, such as that shown in Figure 3, is also a warning sign, even when the activity level is stable. It shows that you are very close to the limit of what your illness will tolerate. If you end up doing a bit more than you had planned for, the road to a relapse is very short. You may well be able to reduce the symptom level by reducing the activity level a few notches, if the high symptom level is caused by overactivity. If the symptoms have other causes, then you should try to remove the other causes. It may still be wise to do a little less for a period as well, to avoid overloading your body until it is better balanced again.

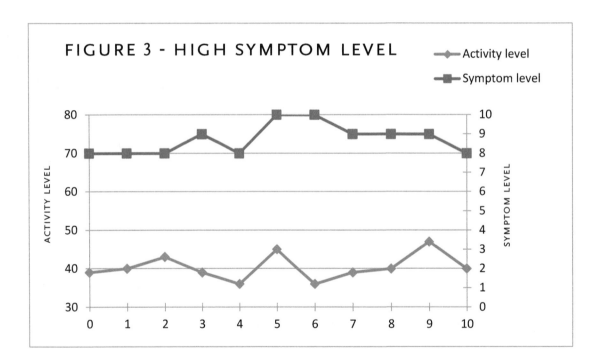

INCREASING SYMPTOM LEVEL, UNSTABLE ACTIVITY LEVEL

The first sign that the illness is worsening is usually that the symptom level increases. This is shown in Figure 4. After a while the condition becomes more unstable (see Figures 1 and 6). In the end the symptom level gets so high that you are forced to do less and less.

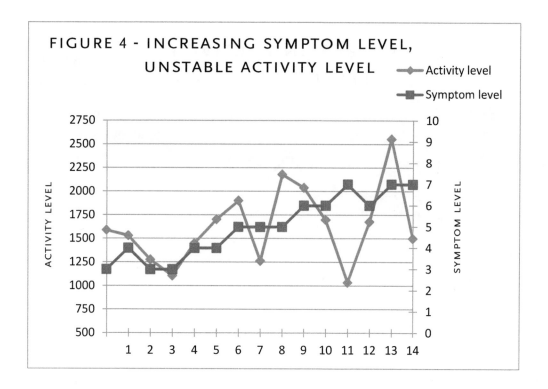

A DECREASING ACTIVITY LEVEL

Both an increasing symptom level and a declining activity level can occur over a time period of a few days or over many months. No matter which of them you observe, you should quickly take steps to stop the decrease and attempt to stabilise the condition in order to feel better. Necessary steps are described in Chapter 8, 'Relapses', and in Chapter 11, 'Three Stages – Three Management Strategies'. A decreasing activity level can be seen in Figure 5.

FALSE IMPROVEMENT

On the basis of the activity level in Figure 6 it looks as though the patient is in steady improvement. The problem is that the symptom level is steadily increasing too. Increasing the activity level steadily without taking the symptom level into consideration will not lead to improvement. This is, in fact, a sure way to provoke a serious relapse. If activity increase leads to worsening of symptoms, you should wait before you increase.

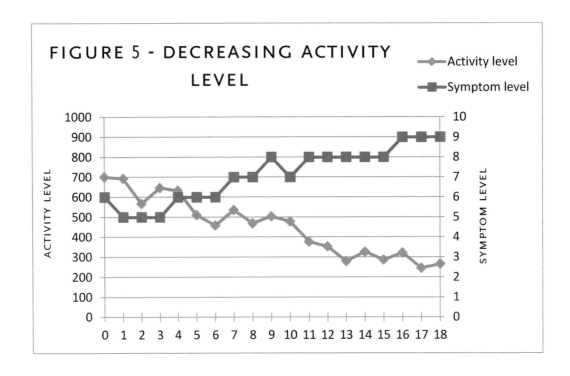

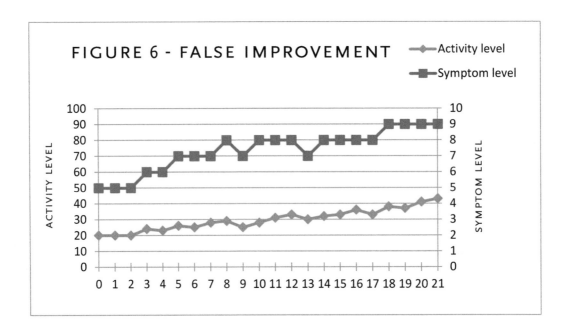

SUDDEN INCREASE

Figure 7 shows one of the classic mistakes. Here the person has been stable for a while and the symptom level has gone down. Then the person thinks that it is possible to do a lot more because the symptoms have gone down. The person increases the activity level abruptly. Best case scenario, this slows down or stops the improvement. Worst case, this ends with a relapse, and the person has to start all over again from the bottom. Even when you feel much better it is important to increase gradually and carefully. How you can do this is described in Chapter 7. A similar pattern to that in Figure 7 can also develop if you increase gradually, but too quickly. Then, after a while you will reach a point where you cannot increase more without becoming more ill. The solution is to cut back for a little while and wait until the symptoms improve. When the improvement of the symptoms is well underway you can increase gradually again. Still you should increase more slowly than before so that the whole thing does not stop abruptly.

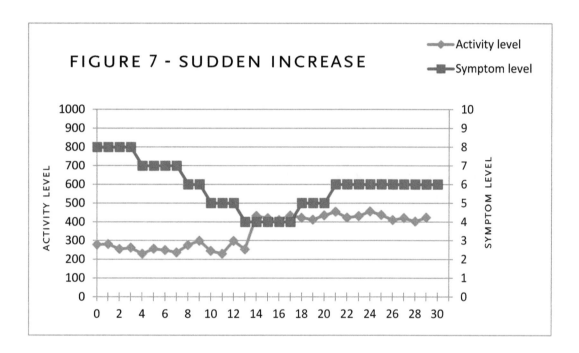

HIGH PEAKS

When you are stable you may find that you can sometimes do far more than usual without getting a relapse afterwards. The pattern that you see in Figure 8 is a good sign. The pattern shows that you are beginning to build up a certain amount of surplus energy. You should not, though, use up this surplus too often. If the high peaks get too close to each other they can slow down the improvement process. If your health does not improve but your condition is pretty stable, it is worth looking at whether frequent high peaks could be holding you back. You should have a goal of having few high peaks in the course of a year, for example four or six. That way you avoid eating away at your surplus energy.

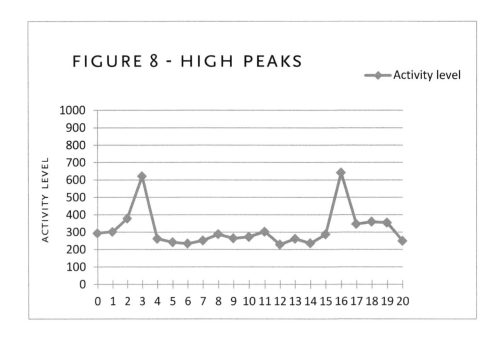

FIGURE 8 - HIGH PEAKS

OVERVIEW OF GOOD PATTERNS

STABILISING

When you stabilise an unstable activity level, it will look similar to Figure 9. In this example the patient stabilises around the bottom of the unstable activity level. By lowering the activity level in this way you will probably get a faster and steadier improvement than if you stabilise at a higher activity level. Chapter 11 describes in detail techniques to help stabilise.

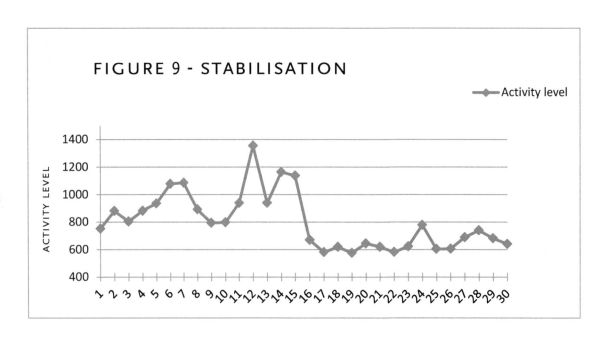

FIGURE 9 - STABILISATION

IMPROVING SYMPTOMS

The first sign of improvement is that the symptom level begins to go down.

The pattern that is seen in Figure 10 is caused by keeping the activity level stable and within your limits for a period of time. Improvement of symptoms can also be due to other causes. It is important to let the symptom level go down a step or so before you attempt to increase the activity level, because this helps to avoid relapse.

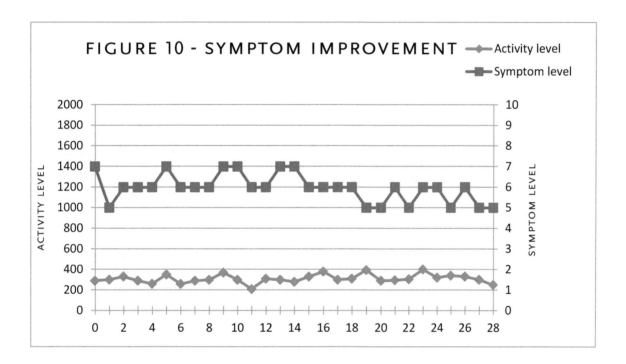

INCREASING ACTIVITY WITH DECLINING SYMPTOM LEVEL

After a while the symptom improvement may pick up speed. Then you can increase the activity level very slowly and carefully without slowing improvement. This pattern shows in Figure 11.

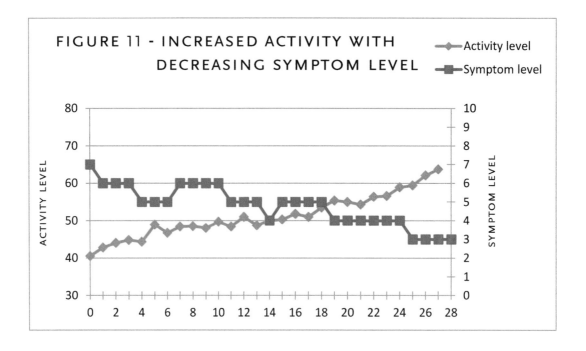

INCREASING ACTIVITY WITH STABLE SYMPTOM LEVEL

If you increase the activity level a bit too fast, there is a risk of the symptom improvement stopping, as you can see in Figure 12.

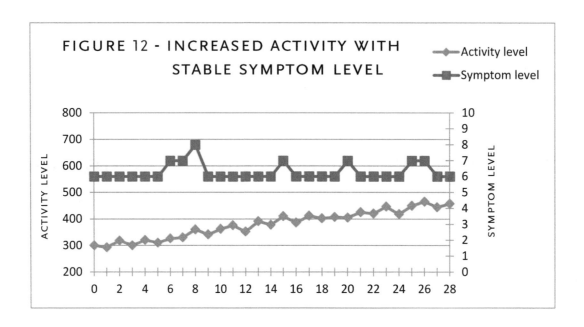

This is not a bad pattern, but in the long run it will feel unsatisfactory that you do not feel better, even if you can do more. It is wise to increase more slowly so that the symptom improvement continues, partially in order to avoid frustration and partially to avoid relapse. Chapter 7 describes how to increase activity in a safe way.

IDEAL IMPROVEMENT CURVE

Figure 13 shows a graph of ideal improvement. This is what the graph shows: First the unstable activity level is stabilised at a low level that does not give symptom increase, either during the course of the same day or in the long run. Then the activity level is kept stable while the symptom level goes down. After a while the improvement gets faster and then the activity level can increase faster. This graph is a schematic example and is not a graph from an actual diary.

This development in an illness is not seen very often, though it does sometimes occur. The norm is that people have big or small relapses along the way, with numerous causes. The reason this graph is included is that it can be useful to have a picture in your mind of what you are aiming for, even though you know that it will not necessarily look this way. It does not matter if the graph ends up looking very different. That is what happens to most of us, including those who experience significant improvement.

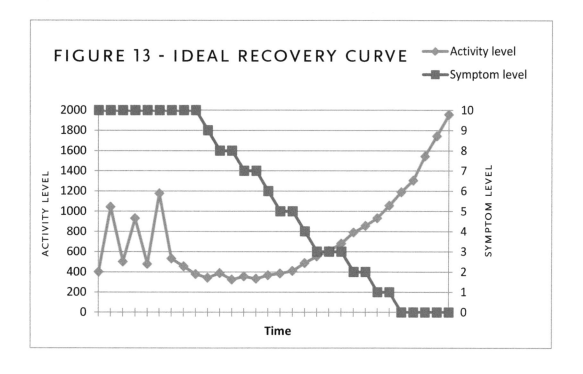

****

Monitoring and interpreting at the macro level is a useful tool no matter whether you make a graph over short or long periods. In Chapter 6 another useful tool is described, namely how to make a flexible routine. That type of routine makes it easier to get as much out of the day as you can, and at the same time get enough rest. With a routine it also becomes easier to keep your activity level stable, which again makes it easier to reach the good patterns that are described in this chapter. Draw a graph from your diary. Find out which of the patterns in this chapter you have right now. Do not get upset if you have one of the unfortunate ones. Most of us have those at times. You can use your diary as an aid to changing the present pattern to a better one that, with a bit of luck, may put you on a path towards gradual improvement.

TASKS

1 Draw a graph where both the activity level and the symptom level are on the same graph.

2 Study the graph and look for these things:

- Which activity level worsens symptoms?

- Which activity level leads to improvement of symptoms?

- Are there patterns that repeat themselves?

- If you have read Chapter 11, which stage are you at?

- Read your activity diary too, so that you can identify reasons for peaks and troughs in both activity and symptom level.

3 See if the graph is similar to any of the patterns described in this chapter.

4 Think about what changes are needed to keep the activity level stable and the symptom level as low as possible.

SUMMARY OF CHAPTER 17

1. Even though ME can make it difficult or impossible to go to school in the normal way, it is often possible to put together an adapted arrangement that makes it possible to get an education.

2. Split all school work into so small spells that you avoid symptom increase. It is better to work for five minutes a day with a clear head, than to do it for a half an hour with a head full of porridge.

3. There are solutions to be found if you have problems reading, writing or doing maths.

4. Home education can be adapted to the pupil's needs. Usually the same goes for online studies.

5. If you are well enough to try to go to school again, it is best to start with just one lesson a week. Do what you can to encourage a good dialogue with the school about adjustments. The school is bound by law to make necessary adjustments to their teaching arrangements.

CHAPTER 17:

LEARNING, SCHOOL AND STUDIES

INTRODUCTION

Going to school and studying is a challenge for children and young people with ME, because everything is set up for people who are healthy. That does not mean that you cannot get an education when you have ME. With the right type of adjustments many will manage to succeed in getting an education. If you have severe ME, you are too ill for formal education and should give priority to looking after your health, instead of pushing yourself with studying that you cannot actually manage. You do not, though, have to climb very far up the functional ability scale before some form of studying can be a part of a varied activity menu. Jane Colby is a former head teacher, and now the leader of The Young ME Sufferer's Trust. She has more than twenty years' experience of advising students, parents and teachers on education and ME.

> Colby points out that: *"Managing a case of childhood ME is not the same as managing an adult case, because children have to be educated by law and inappropriate educational methods can undermine the doctor's management. However, good educational management can be combined with good medical management so that they become two sides of the same coin. Academic success, so far as health and ability permits, can thereby be achieved without provoking further deterioration in the child's condition. This gives an enormous boost to confidence and self-esteem and also helps the child obtain qualifications for the future."*

The advice in this chapter is for both pupils and teachers.

RIGHTS

As a pupil or student you have rights which are defined by law. One of these rights is the right to a suitable education. If you have a medical certificate you have a number of options. It is a good idea to find out what you are entitled to. If you live in the United Kingdom, Tymes Trust can be of help (see the list at the back of the book). If you live in other countries, your national ME charities usually have relevant information material and advisory services. It is useful to have a good dialogue with the school leadership, because they can make sure the teacher follows you up better.

TEACHING MUST BE PACED

The biggest challenge in teaching and ME is that your head gets so tired, even after a very short time. When I did maths as a child it went fine to begin with. I thought it was easy and fun. However, after a quarter of an hour my head was so tired that I could not understand the problems I had solved easily just moments before. There is no point in continuing when you are so tired that you cannot understand the curriculum. You learn nothing in that situation. The teaching situation just makes you feel defeated. Teaching and studying has to be paced. That does not mean that you go on until you no longer grasp what you are doing. It means you stop before you get any symptom increase.

I would probably have got more out of three spells a day of five minutes, than out of one of fifteen minutes. Many people think there is no point in doing lessons if you cannot keep it up for a while. That is a misunderstanding. All music teachers will agree that you get far more out of practising a little every day, than practising a lot one day a week. The same goes for other subjects. Teachers in other subjects are not always aware of this. It is important to remember that a little a day gets to be a lot in the long-run. Five minutes per day is 35 minutes a week and a half hour per day is three and a half hours per week. That turns into a lot of learning in a year. If you are still sceptical, the following example illustrates the point. Three and a half years ago I started listening to a course in Spanish for two to three minutes a day. After three years I had chewed my way through six courses. The last half a year I have listened to audio books intended for people who have had Spanish for two years at school. I have no problems understanding these, even though I still only listen to Spanish for two minutes a day.

FIND THE RIGHT AMOUNT OF TIME FOR LESSONS

Everyone has to experiment to find the right length of time for lessons. You can use Worksheet 1, the experiment sheet that I have described in Chapter 1, or you can make an activity diary as described in Chapter 4. Afterwards you can interpret the results as explained in Chapters 4 and 15. It is quite normal to find that some subjects or study methods take more energy than others. Writing an assignment is often more exhausting than reading or listening. Therefore, it can be a good idea to list separately how long it is sensible to work on the different types of subjects and study activities. When you sit up to do lessons you can check the list and decide for how long you should work. You can use an alarm, for example on your phone, that can ring when it is time to stop.

PLANNING

There are several reasons why it is smart to plan the length of the lessons ahead of time. First of all it means that you will be working with a fairly clear head. Secondly, it means that you stop before your head gets terribly tired or painful. That way you avoid the feeling of defeat that comes with understanding nothing at the end of a session. Thirdly, it is much easier to focus your brain to do lessons when you know that the session will be short and that you will be doing something fun afterwards. Children and young people with ME need a varied daily life with fun, classes and a social life. It is often possible to manage this, but it means that you must do a bit of each and not too much of anything. This needs some planning, which is not always easy with ME. It is easier to do the things you would like, without doing too much, if you have a flexible daily routine. How you can do this is described in Chapter 6. I must emphasise again that people with very severe ME are far too ill to do schoolwork of any type. Jane Colby underlines this: *"Paradoxically, putting education second actually achieves the best education results in this illness."* When you begin to get better, schoolwork can be a part of a varied activity menu without it leading to relapse.

AVOID BEING DISTRACTED

When you have ME, it is very easy to become distracted and therefore you must reduce as many factors that can distract you as possible, so that you can concentrate. Sounds are particularly distracting, so close windows and doors, turn off machines that are not in use, like the radio, TV or computer. Use ear defenders if necessary. Remove flowers that smell and throw away the chewing gum. If you get distracted by things you see, it can help to work at a table that is empty of everything except what you need here and now. It is important that you are not too cold or too hot, hungry or need to go to the toilet. If there are other people in the room it helps to ask them to sit completely still. These measures do not remove concentration problems, but can reduce them just enough that you can manage to work for a short while. Many of these measures are difficult to do in a classroom, which illustrates the importance of adaptive schooling.

THINK ENERGY CONSERVATION

At school it is usual that the pupils are asked to do many tasks and problems of the same type whether they have learned the subject or not. The school goes in for quantity instead of quality. The idea is that all children will, after a while, have learned what is necessary. This is a bad idea for people with ME because it means throwing away energy on things that have already been learned. It is better to identify what you do not know and work specifically on that. Every now and then you can repeat some tasks in subjects you already know, just to keep up the skills. If you systematically prioritise quality before quantity it is amazing how many pupils with ME manage to get through subjects, when they would definitely not have been able to do so if they had had to do it the same way the other pupils do. Jane Colby says:

> *"Processes like brain-storming, drafting and finally producing a finished piece of writing are too exhausting for many children with ME and both their health and the quality of the work will suffer unless the processes required are reduced to a minimum."*

SPECIFIC LEARNING DIFFICULTIES

It is not uncommon for people with ME to get specific learning difficulties when they become ill, according to Siw Jönsson, a Norwegian special education teacher. Specific learning difficulties that can occur are difficulties with listening, speaking and understanding, plus difficulties with mathematics. Often it is a question of either reading or maths difficulties, but you can get both. Some get totally different problems, for example difficulties with speaking. Motor learning difficulties are common. With specific learning difficulties it is extra important to use very short spells of work and to focus on learning the most central and necessary part of the curriculum. In the next paragraphs I give you some tips you can use for different types of learning difficulties.

READING DIFFICULTIES

At school you read for two reasons, partly to practise reading and partly to acquire knowledge in other subjects. When you have a lot of reading problems it can be difficult or almost impossible to acquire knowledge through reading. This, however, does not mean that it is impossible to learn. The curriculum for all school levels is available as audio books. There is therefore no reason to wear yourself out attempting to read difficult texts if it is easier to listen. How audio versions of school books are obtained varies from country to country, but a special education teacher or relevant organisation will know how.

In the book, *A Parent's Guide to CFIDS*, Dr. David Bell and the other authors point out that for some it is easier to remember the contents of an audio book if they follow the lines in the book at the same time. If you have a home tutor, the tutor can, of course, present the material. For some, video is easier than audio books. There are a number of good educational videos and DVDs. A good teacher can help you to find these. Many adults would be surprised to hear that young teachers often use videos from YouTube (www.youtube.com) in their lessons. These might be historical film snippets and documentary films of a high quality, which are often available in short bits. This makes pacing simpler. Still, there is a lot on YouTube that is not appropriate for educational purposes. It takes time and energy to sort out the useful things. It is helpful if the tutor can find good video sources, so that the pupil's energy is saved for more useful projects.

In order to carry out pure reading training you must, of course, read, but you do not need to read a whole book. People with serious reading difficulties will learn more from reading single words or a few sentences than they do by trying to push themselves into reading large amounts of text. When you are well enough to be able to read a block of text you can use notices in newspapers or other texts that are short. It is much easier to read large letters than small, so notices like those mentioned above can be made even larger by magnifying them using a scanner or photocopier. If you get distracted when there is a lot of text on a page, you can use a reading prosthesis. In Chapter 3 I describe how one can be made quite easily. Some feel that it is easier to read if the background colour is not white. You can experiment with other colours by changing the background colour on the computer. There are also special plastic sheets that can be placed on top of written text. These are called coloured overlays and are normally used in dyslexia. You can also get books that are made especially to simplify reading. They have short lines, large letters and double spacing. They are also written in a simple language that is not childish. Therefore, these books are an excellent step towards ordinary books. You might also find standard large-print books easier to read.

DIFFICULTIES WITH WRITING

It is not unusual for people with ME to be unable to write by hand for a long time. Also, some have great problems concentrating when attempting to express themselves in writing. School goals include learning to express oneself in writing. This includes spelling, constructing sentences and writing longer passages. Writing by hand is part of the curriculum. Just as with reading you can work with one part at a time instead of all three at once. You do not have to write to be able to express yourself clearly. This can be learned by dictating, either to a person or a Dictaphone.

You can get computer programs which make it possible to dictate directly to a computer, which then writes down what you say. The English program is called Dragon Naturally Speaking. This program can read the text back to you, and allows you to dictate changes. The more you use it, the better the voice recognition gets. Unfortunately, it is quite expensive. There are also several application programs (apps) that make it possible to dictate to a mobile phone, including a mobile version of Dragon. Many of these are free or cheap. This is an area where developments are quick, so it is difficult to give concrete advice on what to use, except that Dragon is probably better than some of the other programs. The accuracy of the mobile phone dictation programs is not great yet, so you have to read through the text to be sure that the program is writing the correct words. Therefore, these programs are not yet suitable for people with severe reading problems or problems focusing their eyes. Many people feel that it is easier to write using a computer than by hand.

Learning spelling and punctuation does not require writing large amounts of text.

You can learn to spell single words and you can set punctuation marks in texts that someone else has written down. In order to learn handwriting you must, of course, write, but even this can be done in short spells. Pupils with ME should not be given low marks because of ugly handwriting due to poor fine motor skills, which can be part of the illness.

DIFFICULTIES WITH MATHEMATICS

Even with problems with mathematics, it is an advantage to try to define where the problem lies. Concentration problems in ME may often have peculiar consequences, like when I started learning algebra. We were given simplification problems that were simple, but very long. I knew exactly how to solve them, but because they were so long, it was still too much for my head. I could attempt the same problem twice from one direction and once backwards and get three different answers. If I was unlucky, none of the answers were right. After a while we learned more difficult rules like multiplying out brackets. Then the problems were much shorter and I no longer had problems with algebra as long as I did not do too much at a time.

The right kind of problem is, therefore, important for the results. Many people with ME write numbers in the wrong order. Siw Jönsson, a special education teacher, says that it can help if the problems have been written down ahead of time so that you just have to do the maths. If you say a correct number out loud but still end up writing it incorrectly, you can try dictating them while watching someone else write them down. It is difficult to make a reading prosthesis for mathematics. You can, though, use white pieces of paper to cover the problems that you are not working on, so that you do not get distracted. People with ME who have problems with maths often have problems with organisation and logic, which I, too, have experienced.

As a child I could not sort things or straighten up my room. My parents had to teach me how you split things into categories. Later I learned other disciplines that are reminiscent of mathematics, but which do not use numbers, such as grammar and music theory. The odd thing is that the better I got at mathematics without numbers, the easier it was to calculate with numbers, too.

HOME TUITION

Home tuition is the easiest way to adjust teaching to the needs of children with ME. Jane Colby says: *"The goal of education is to educate; where this takes place is secondary to that aim. It should be the place that produces the best results. The most suitable environment for a child suffering with ME is often the home as it involves no expenditure of energy travel."* With home tuition both the length of sessions and the working methods can be tailored to the needs of the pupil. It is necessary to remember that even being taught at home is tiring for people with more severe ME. Siw Jönsson points out that instruction should wait until the pupil is well enough to receive knowledge. The educational psychology office in Kongsberg and Numedal in Norway is experienced in adapting education to the needs of children with ME. They write:

> *"When pupils are weak from ME there is little point in instruction. We have seen that home tuition for some pupils is not desirable, while in others it is absolutely necessary. The office has seen that the severity of the illness varies individually, so that every pupil who experiences the exhaustion/has the diagnosis needs individually adapted measures. Therefore, evaluation is necessary in order to decide whether the pupil is able to receive instruction, and it is also necessary to evaluate the intensity, frequency and content in the light of their abilities and qualifications."*

Many pupils, parents and teachers feel that it is hard and difficult to have to put off education for a period. It is important to underline that formal education is something one can receive at any age. If pausing your education helps your health, the pause is not wasted.

Jane Colby points out that it is important to avoid rollercoaster education, where the pupil attempts school full-time or considerably more lessons during good periods and then collapses. If you increase studying gradually even when improvement is abrupt, there is a greater chance that the increase will not lead to overactivity and result in relapse. This applies no matter what kind of studying you are doing.

It is important that the teacher gets proper information about ME. Most ME organisations can usually give you good information meant for teachers. One of the most important things a home tutor can do is to focus on the main points in the curriculum, since the pupil with ME is most likely not able to take in all the details. It is better to have a good grasp of the main points, and miss some of the detail, than knowing the details of one part of the subject, and nothing about the rest of it. Once you have the main points, it is easy to collect the details when you are well enough or need them. This is confirmed by Jane Colby, who writes:

> *"For the best results it is necessary to follow, not a broad and balanced curriculum, but a focused one, concentrating on a few subjects and minimising course-work. This leads to real achievement in those subjects. Achievement is the child's entitlement. It raises morale and demonstrates that real success is possible."*

The greatest advantage of home schooling is that the lessons can be tailored to the pupil's needs. You do not have to be able to manage a session lasting 45 minutes. Instead, you can split up the lessons into one or more short sessions with rest breaks in between. During the rest breaks the teacher can correct homework or plan the next session. When you are well enough to keep going for 45 minutes, you can save a lot of energy by switching between practical and theoretical work. It can also be a good idea to switch between different subjects and different ways of working – listening, reading, writing, problem solving etc. Teachers are used to thinking along traditional lines. You cannot be sure that the teacher will see that it can be a good idea to carry out lessons in a different way. It is important to have good communication between pupil, parents and teacher. The teacher needs to understand the advantages of adjusting the teaching to the pupil's state of health. Not only does the pupil learn more, but the pupil will also benefit in terms of their health and symptom levels.

Home tuition is an effective way of learning. A girl who had home tuition at high school level told me that she learned as much during one lesson as her classmates learned in a week. The girl did not have many lessons a week but got through almost all the subjects. It is good to know that you do not need to reach a normal functioning level to be able to keep up with your classmates academically.

GOING TO SCHOOL PART-TIME

The first question of interest when it comes to part-time schooling is how well you have to be to be able to go to school now and then. The American paediatrician David Bell has found that being in a shopping centre is about as demanding as going to school. If you can manage two hours at a shopping centre, you can probably manage two hours at school. You should not attempt part-time school if you are ill for several hours or days after being in a shopping centre for an hour. Then it's better to choose home tuition or other forms of home education for now. When you try part-time schooling the first time after having been away, you should start off with an hour once a week to begin with.

Jill Moss is a former head of a centre for special education at a mainstream secondary school and started the Association of Young People with ME. She recommends that you first and foremost choose a lesson that happens at a time of day when you do not feel too bad and a subject that you like. When you are well enough to increase, it's probably better to choose a lesson another day than to attempt to do two lessons in the same day. At secondary school level it is best to increase subject by subject, which means that when you are able to increase you add another lesson in the same subject and postpone other subjects until you can attend all lessons in the subject you first started. Once you can manage all the lessons in the first subject, you can start building up a second subject in the same way if your health permits. This is because it is better to succeed at taking exams in one subject than it is to try several subjects and maybe not manage any of them.

Some schools group their lessons so that you have several lessons in the same subject on the same day. If they do it that way at your school, then you have to consider what is best for you – is it better to take a lesson in a different subject on a separate day, or to have consecutive lessons in the same subject? Jill Moss underlines that in primary/elementary school and at the intermediate level it can be an advantage to join different lessons instead of taking just one subject. Yet this must be evaluated in each case. It is not always easy to take part in only one weekly lesson in a subject.

Not all teachers make sure that you get to know what has happened in the lessons you could not join. The teachers do not always make sure that part-time students get the books and materials that the rest of the class received. In my early teens I had a super German teacher who made weekly plans, so that I could see what the class had been doing while I was gone. Even when the rest of the class did not get a plan, she made one for me. None of the other teachers could be bothered. Several times I found I had come to a maths lesson unprepared for a test that the others had been told about in the lessons when I was absent, and it seemed as though the teachers felt that if I could not come to all the lessons, it was my problem. This underlines how important good communication with teachers is. It is important to explain what you need, and it is not unreasonable to ask to be made aware of what goes on when one is unable to be there.

It is not a good idea to be too ambitious at the beginning of the school year and then crash. When you plan the next school year you should take as a starting point what you can do now, and not what you hope you can do in the autumn. If your health improves over the summer you should still start carefully and increase gradually only if you can manage it. The school is usually happy to hear that you can do more than you thought, but it can be more difficult to have to cut back on school time. I am aware of a number of kids who seemed fully recovered but who still relapsed badly when they tried a full course load at school. When you increase gradually, you will be able to put the brakes on in time if you feel that you have reached the limit of what you can do. This can prevent relapse.

ENERGY CONSERVATION AT SCHOOL

School can be a very exhausting place to be. Jill Moss says:

> *"Stressful environments draw on our meagre supplies of energy before we even think about carrying a heavy bag around and sitting up for an extended period on a hard chair, or even worse, a science stool! All this and the brain hasn't even started listening to and assimilating information."*

Luckily there are a number of energy economising initiatives that can make the school day simpler both for part-time and full-time pupils. In some places it is possible to ask to sit in a quiet corner or a group room. In some situations ear defenders can help. A comfortable chair may also help. In some countries, this can be borrowed from the national health service. You can find out more about aids in Chapter 23, 'Tips for Energy Conservation'. A laptop computer can make writing simpler. A key to the elevator and an electric wheelchair or scooter can make it possible to move around the school with the other pupils. If you get two sets of books you will not have to carry them back and forth between home and school. A school assistant can help you move equipment and push your wheelchair. The assistant can also assist you with things that have to do with cognitive functions, for example keeping your appointments and lessons straight, checking that you are bringing the right books home with you. It is smart to ask the school whether they have a place where you can lie down and rest. When you are well enough to manage more than one lesson a day, it is easier if you can rest for an hour before you take another lesson. Universities usually have such rest rooms, often in connection with the toilets.

EXAMS

One of the most important adaptations that can help you during exams when you have ME, is to avoid overexertion beforehand. If you read much more than usual, you risk getting a relapse, and worse case can become too ill to take exams. It is usually better to stick to your normal routine and perhaps add a little extra rest. If you are nervous about not managing to revise everything, it can help to learn more about study techniques to help you prioritise your time in the lead-up to the exam. Techniques for stress management can also help. Most student associations offer psychological help in managing exams, and school counsellors may also be able to help.

There are a number of other things you can do, and concessions you could apply for to make exams easier. You can get extra time and rest breaks, and also permission to use a computer for writing instead of writing by hand. At some places, including universities, it is possible to ask for a different form of exam, instead of a written exam. You must check the deadline for applying for concessions in connection with exams. This is usually several months before the exam. The application must be accompanied by a doctor's certificate. In some countries, doctor's certificates for concessions are only valid for one year, so do check the rules in your country.

ONLINE STUDIES

Online studies are suitable for many people with ME because you can work from home at your own pace. Availability varies from country to country, but often, most levels are available. If you are still within statutory school age and use online studies or other correspondence courses as an alternative to home tuition, you may get funding for this. Young people with ME in Australia say that part-time correspondence is very well suited for people with ME, but that full-time correspondence, if anything, is more work than full-time school. At high school level, both theoretical and vocational courses are usually available, but vocational courses may involve one or more placements. I have heard of people who were able to negotiate getting the diploma without having done the placement because they were too ill, but this may not always be possible. When it comes to higher education, there is also a wide range of courses available, but some courses may be too specialised to be available. Be aware that some online studies have weekend seminars where you meet up with fellow students for intensive studying. Intensive courses like this can be much more exhausting than taking a course for example one day a week. In some countries people who receive state benefits may get distance learning courses for free. Online courses from private educational establishments may be very expensive. Exam concessions and other adaptations are usually available even in distance-learning environments. Be sure to enquire about this before signing up for the course.

MASSIVE OPEN ONLINE COURSES

In recent years, a new type of online course has appeared, so-called *massive open online courses (MOOCs)*, which are free online courses run by high-profile universities. These are typically available through private companies, some of which are for profit and some of which are non-profit. MOOCs are usually available in two forms. One is entirely free and gives no formal qualifications, the other type costs a bit of money but offers a certificate to prove that you completed the course. Certificates typically cost 50 to 100 US dollars. There is no formal exam at the end; instead you pass the course by passing all graded assignments. Because of the lack of exam, free courses do not weigh as heavily as formal university courses, but doing one or more of these still shows that you are motivated to learn. The smallest courses require two to four hours a week, but larger courses may require up to twelve hours of work per week.

Each of the MOOC companies offers courses from a variety of subjects. There appears to be a particularly good range of computer science and business courses, but you can find just about anything. However, each company's collection of courses within a subject often appears arbitrary. You may, for instance, find three specialized psychology courses from different universities, but no basic information about the subject. You may well have to search the websites of several companies to find what you want. If you go to Wikipedia and search for Massive Open Online Courses, or Free Online Courses, you will get a list of relevant companies. Free online courses are useful if you are unsure whether you are well enough for formal studying, because they enable you to try studying without the risk of losing lots of money if you cannot complete the course.

HIGHER EDUCATION

All colleges and universities have a contact person or a consultant service for people with disabilities. The consultant knows which adaptions are possible and, if necessary, can advocate for you if necessary. You should contact this person as soon as possible, preferably before you start your studies. Do not wait until you run into problems. It is easier to prevent problems from occurring than to solve them when they turn up.

In higher education the courses are set up in different ways. Many university courses have few lectures and lots of time when you study on your own. Courses like these are good for people with ME because it is less exhausting to do your studying at home or in a reading room than attending a lecture. Study progression is often better than when studying a subject that has a full timetable. It is, though, an advantage to study part-time so you can have a more balanced life and not just study all the time. It is easier to avoid relapses if you have different activities in your timetable.

Some professional subjects at colleges and universities have a heavy timetable and long periods of practice, where you are expected to work more or less full-time and study on the side. This can be very difficult for people with ME, but some of these subjects may be found as part-time courses, too. With any course, it is worth contacting the person responsible for accessibility ahead of time to find out which adaptations can be made.

Students also have to consider their financial situation. Many countries have arrangements for student loans or scholarships, education grants etc. There may also be special education financial grants for disabled students. Check out your options ahead of time. If you are able to work a little, it might be possible to take courses in connection with the job, sometimes even paid by your employer. If you receive social security benefits, or suchlike, find out whether the studying you would like to do might lead to changes in the amount you are receiving. Check the rules and ask for them in writing.

****

When everything is chaos and your head is full of porridge, it is easy to think that education is a remote dream that can never come true. Luckily, careful pacing can make your illness more stable and lessen your symptoms, so that education can become realistic. Using the advice in this chapter, many people are able to put together an education even though it often takes longer when you have ME.

TASKS

1 Consider whether you are well enough to study and which type of education would be suitable for you.

2 Think through the cognitive problems you have. Make a list of them. Think about which adaptations you may need.

3 Choose the energy conservation measures that are best for you.

SUMMARY OF CHAPTER 18

1. In severe ME, the slightest stimulation, thought or movement must be counted as activity.

2. To stabilise when you have severe ME you must reduce your activity level drastically. It can be necessary to take total rest and extreme steps like tube-feeding to relieve the pressure on your body.

3. People with severe ME have very tight limits. A few minutes of extra activity can lead to serious relapse.

4. Physical rest is not enough. You must learn to switch off mentally too. This can make the difference between getting better and not getting better.

5. There are a number of ways to obtain some quality of life with severe ME. If you use these it will be easier to endure the situation until your health improves.

CHAPTER 18:

SEVERE ME

INTRODUCTION

Pacing is always challenging, but it is extra challenging when you are bed-bound or too ill to go out. The reason for this is that people with severe ME often no longer have many activities to cut down on. That makes it harder to get enough healing rest. The rest of this chapter could have been filled with suggestions for energy conservation that make activities like eating and going to the toilet easier, and, by using them, increase the amount of healing rest.

That, though, is not the object of this chapter. Nor is it a guide to nursing people with severe ME, although relatives and assistants are likely to find reading this chapter useful. Instead, we will look at how to pace activities when you are so ill that everything is really too much. If you need general information on living with severe ME I suggest you read Jodi Basset's, *Caring for the ME Patient*, and Claire Wade's, *Surviving Severe ME*. You can also read Emily Collingridge's *Severe ME/CFS: A Guide to Living*. See the reference list for more information. It is normal for people with severe ME to have a greatly reduced tolerance to sensory input. Tips on how to tackle this can be found at the back of the book.

GRASP THE SEVERITY — BE DRASTIC

When you get severe ME it can often take a little time before you understand how ill you actually are. This is unfortunate because it often means that you end up doing too much. For example, you might go out, despite the fact that you are exhausted after having put on your shoes and jacket. Another example is choosing to lie down on the sofa despite the fact that you have to have rest breaks on several different chairs in order to get there, and you are still exhausted when you finally arrive. When we say that people with ME should stay inside their limits, it means that you do not go out if you are exhausted by putting on your jacket. In the same way you stay in bed if you get worn out by trying to reach the sofa. It is alright to experiment with placing an armchair beside your bed to see if you can sit in it for a short period without getting more ill. If you cannot manage that, it is best to stay in bed. In the same way you do not have to wash every day if it is exacerbating your symptoms, or eat at a table, or eat with a knife and fork. You can be fed, or drink soup or purée (mashed food) with a straw. Nor do you need to go all the way out to the toilet if it is too exhausting or painful. It is possible to put a commode beside the bed or use a bedpan or urinal bottle. This sort of arrangement is often felt to be very drastic and frightening.

Many people wait far too long before choosing to use this sort of measure. As mentioned in Chapter 10, the amount of healing rest can make the difference between deterioration and improvement. In order for severe ME to improve you usually have to use this type of strategy. It is far better to start using them right away and maybe only need to use them for a few weeks, rather than trying to resist for a long time, and get even more ill from doing too much. You can often avoid becoming so ill that you are totally dependent on care if you rest enough at the start of an acute relapse. The Norwegian doctor Sidsel Kreyberg points out that both active and passive activity may give symptom increase, and this proves the importance of enough rest. It is normal for people with severe ME to lose functional ability in one or more body parts. How you use healing rest to help bring back your functional ability is discussed in Chapter 12, 'Challenges in pacing'.

Drastic measures should be used to get enough rest, not as a means to use your energy as much as possible. The reason for this is that there is a great risk of relapse when the condition is unstable, and even small overexertions lead to great consequences. Zoë Williams, who has had severe ME for many years, says:

> *"When you are very ill, it is a matter of survival, even small mistakes in pacing can lead to horrible consequences."*

MENTAL REST

When you already spend your day in bed it can be difficult to increase the amount of physical rest. That makes it even more important to have mental rest, too. People with severe ME are often so weak that even simple thought processes drain them totally. The occupational therapist Irma Pinxterhuis found this in connection with her study of people with very severe ME. Sidsel Kreyberg has also pointed this out. It can be difficult for your body to recover without mental rest. So you must make sure to pace all mental activities carefully so that they do not lead to an increase in your symptoms. This includes pleasant activities like TV, audio books, reading, computer use, and talking, even if this means that you are bored for part of the day. People with severe ME can feel mentally overstimulated – they get 'wired'. You can read more about this in Chapter 12, 'Challenges in Pacing'. It can be difficult to relax, too, when you have strong physical symptoms. This makes it a good idea to learn relaxation techniques that can help you 'switch off'. In Chapter 3, 'Cognitive Activities', there are instructions for a relaxation session you can try and at the back of the book there is a list of relaxation resources. British patients who have been hospitalised in specialist clinics for severely ill ME patients, often say that the hardest thing in hospital was learning relaxation. Even if it is difficult, it can be an essential key to improvement.

In the article *Rest and Relaxation for Recovery*, Kathryn D. wrote:

> *"Have you ever felt that you are not resting, even if you do nothing but rest? Have you ever wanted to relax more but feel your body just can't let go, and your mind won't stop racing? Rest, relaxation and letting go have been very important in lifting me out of many years of being severely ill. I changed subtly something inside that made a big difference to my body being able to fully rest and recuperate. I had been in bed, too ill to get up, for five years. I finally, purposefully, let go inside. Before, I didn't realise how important it was – I finally felt able to rest fully."*

Here, we see that Kathryn managed to 'let go inside', that is switch off completely, empty her head, give herself permission to rest completely and to follow her body's needs, instead of fighting the illness all the time. That was when she got deeper rest.

All forms of relaxation demand a degree of concentration. It is common for people with severe ME to feel that certain types of relaxation are too demanding. Yet there are often one or more types of relaxation that work well or that can be used in given situations. So do not give up if the first type turns out to be unsuitable. Perhaps the least demanding kind of relaxation is to sigh at the same time as you relax your muscles. This exercise takes only two seconds and needs almost no concentration – yet it releases muscle tension and can therefore reduce pain. Some people feel this exercise is useful in making it easier to cope with personal care, which is uncomfortable, but necessary.

If real relaxation exercises are too exhausting, you can actually experience a certain degree of relaxation by thinking quiet thoughts. When you are overstimulated and find it difficult to calm down you can deliberately choose to think about lovely landscapes or anything else you associate with peacefulness and pleasure. If you find that relaxation is not good for you, do not use the technique. When ME patients feel that a method is not working for them, it is important that they must not feel pressured into using it. People with ME are capable of evaluating what works for them, even when they have a very reduced ability to communicate.

There is another reason why it is important to learn mental rest. Many of those with ME have experienced getting stressed or overstimulated by small things that never stressed them before they became ill, even by fun activities. This is often a symptom of ME, and people find that it improves when the ME improves. It can be a good idea to mention this to those around you so they do not think that the sensitivity to stress is a part of your personality. Being stressed or overstimulated takes a lot of energy. A young woman who has had very severe ME told me that it had been very useful for her to choose not to care about certain things, such as when a personal assistant slightly confused her routine, instead of using all her energy on being stressed. This is not a miracle cure, but it can help give you a little more energy in your everyday life.

VERY NARROW LIMITS

Those with severe ME have very precise and restricted limits both physically and mentally. Even the slightest amount of sensory input, thinking or movement must be considered activity, and even this little can be far too much. Even a couple of minutes of cheering small talk from your assistants or family can be so demanding that it often hinders improvement or leads to deterioration. The difference between a sustainable level of activity and overdoing it can be the difference between swallowing once and doing it twice in a row, or the difference between shifting slightly and turning over in bed. In this situation it is obvious that it is not possible to always manage to stay within one's limits. There are, for example, times when one must say two sentences even when you can really only manage one. This kind of overexertion has nothing to do with lack of self-discipline. It has to do with the severity of the illness, and the fact that meeting one's needs is not simple at this level. People who think that it is always possible to avoid this kind of overexertion are both unreasonable and ignorant. These small overexertions are one of the factors that means severe ME can last a long time. It is simply not as easy for people who are severely ill to get healing rest as it is for people who are less ill.

In order to get healing rest there are two things you must do. First of all you must make sure to limit the activities that actually can be limited and which you have control over. That way you have more energy left to tackle the small overexertions that you cannot prevent. For someone with severe ME, splitting things into small enough sessions can mean that one part of your body gets washed one day and another part the next day, or the week after. Changing clothes, having meals etc., can be split into very small chunks too. One patient found that her health started to improve when she began to rest for ten minutes between every bite of food she took when eating.

Secondly, you have to make sure you get several long, deep rest breaks during which you actually get healing rest. When I was at my worst I had to lie absolutely still for two hours before my body got warm. Sometimes my feet never warmed up, even if I kept them up against a hot water bottle. As soon as I moved I got cold again. It was my experience that circulation was very important for healing rest, so I chose a strategy where I attempted to split all activities into such small bits that I did not get cold, and I also rested for so long that I got warm again every time I had the chance. This strategy led to many years of gradual and accelerating improvement.

STABILISING

Many people with ME have confusing fluctuations both in their level of functioning and symptom level. In Chapter 11, I describe how you can encourage stabilisation of symptoms by stabilising the activity level. The advice in that chapter is also suitable for people with severe ME. If you have severe ME it is extra important to have structure to your day. You may find that you have such great problems with your concentration and memory that you have trouble structuring your own day, or even with remembering how long you can safely do activities. It can help to have a relatively regular routine where daily tasks such as meals and personal hygiene are spread out at set times with sufficient rests in between. This way you can accomplish pacing without having to think so much.

To maintain stability, and hopefully eventual improvement, it is very important that you stick to the routine even on good days. You must not fall for the temptation to do more. Many with severe ME have such narrow limits that just doing five minutes extra of something can lead to lasting consequences. The advice on not doing more on a good day can be extra difficult to follow for people with severe ME. Often it is only on the good days that one can be washed or do/experience something nice. Still, it is helpful to try to restrain yourself as much as possible, to try and avoid the rollercoaster pattern described in Chapter 16. That pattern can get in the way of improvement.

The purpose of stabilising the condition is to get the dramatic symptoms under control and get the general symptoms down to a tolerable level. When you have had a high symptom level for a long time it is a relief to find the worst symptoms reduced. Despite this, one is often left with a symptom level that is so high that it is not advisable to increase the activity level.

If you have a bad memory it can be useful to ask those around you to remind you that you must save your energy on good days. Those around you may also find it useful to be reminded that you are not well enough to do more even if you seem a bit better. It is only when the stabilisation is well-established that you should attempt to do a little bit more on a good day. Even then it is best to ensure that the extra activity is so small that it does not entail symptom increase. You could for example have a rule that you either do something pleasant like looking at a picture, or something useful like having you hair brushed, but not both.

Stabilisation often takes a long time in severe ME. You must not get impatient and attempt to force an improvement by increasing activity; unfortunately this will only lead to relapse. If, though, you find a daily routine that functions with a minimum of symptom flaring and discomfort, and make sure of getting several rest breaks with healing rest each day then improvement will often come of itself. In Chapters 6 and 15 there are examples of parts of routines for both severe and very severe ME. These can be used as inspiration, but must, of course, be adjusted to suit each individual. The examples may not be suitable at all.

THE FIRST SIGNS OF IMPROVEMENT

In the beginning the improvement process will usually go very slowly. The first signs of improvement may be, for example, that you have the energy to say two sentences one after another, or that you manage to turn over in bed without getting exhausted. It could also be that you notice that it has been many weeks since you had a very bad day. At this stage there are two things that are very important.

The first is that you must try not to get over-enthusiastic and think that you can do a lot more. When the improvement process is moving slowly the body needs all that available surplus to heal itself. It is far too early to increase deliberately. The small, spontaneous increases that are difficult to avoid doing are enough. These sorts of increases are things like scratching oneself, brushing hair away from your face, or focussing your eyes for longer. It can be very difficult to avoid doing things like this when you feel you have the energy, even if it might be better to save it for something more important later. With improvement you are almost certain to be increasing these sorts of activity naturally, which is why it is best to wait a while before you increase other things deliberately. This is so you do not use up the healing rest and, by doing so, stop the improvement. Hang on to the main focus: it is healing rest that creates the improvement. Medical input can also have a good effect (for example medication for pain or sleep, or tube feeding), but unfortunately not everyone with ME has access to suitable medical care.

The second thing to think about is registering the small steps forward as they occur. Dictate them, perhaps, to an assistant and get the person to write them down with the date or do it yourself if this is simpler. When the advances come very slowly it is easy to become disheartened and feel that you are not getting better at all. On days like those you may find it encouraging to get someone to read the list of the small improvements to you.

MOTIVATION INCREASES

Spontaneous increases are typically about everyday activities like eating, using the toilet, and important messages. Even though it is pleasant to experience managing more of this, it is not especially inspiring in the long run. Then it might be the right time to try something called motivation increases. Motivation increases should not be attempted before the improvement process is well-established. These are tiny, deliberate increases that are introduced exclusively for enjoyment. The increase should be so tiny that they do not lead to symptom increase. In the beginning you should not attempt motivation increases more often than every third month, and even after a while you should not do it more often than every second month. The purpose of the motivation increases is to have something pleasant to do so that you can endure the waiting time until you are well enough to increase at a quicker tempo. It is not always easy to find activities that suit people with very severe ME. In Figure 1 I have listed some of the activity suggestions Zoë Williams has presented in her collection of tips for ME patients.

FIGURE 1 – NON-DEMANDING ACTIVITIES

From www.metips.co.uk

- Watch someone blowing bubbles

- Put on a temporary tattoo

- Use a scented candle (not for those with sensitivity to smell)

- Meditate or do relaxation exercises

- Get a helium balloon that is nice to look at

- Close your eyes and think of a lovely place

- Look at clouds or stars

- Eat good food and perhaps try some new and exciting recipes

OTHER SUGGESTIONS:

- Look at a picture of something you like, i.e. a beautiful landscape

- Taste something delicious

- Read or dictate a text message

- Watch seeds and plants sprout and grow

- Listen to a poem from an audio book (there are poems of less than 30 seconds)

- Decorate a card with a sticker per day

Many with ME find that daily life can seem monotonous. Virtual holidays (pretend vacations) and virtual parties can be a way of obtaining variation. Virtual holidays and parties are about imagining you are on vacation or at a party. On top of day-dreaming you can look at pictures from the place where you are 'vacationing', eat a meal from that area, hear or read something about the area and whatever else you can think of which you are well enough to do. You can decide how much you want to make of it and do any other connected activities spread across the following days. You can read more about virtual holidays in Chapter 19, 'Social activities'.

WHEN THE PROCESS OF IMPROVEMENT IS WELL UNDER WAY

It is only when the illness is improving so quickly that it is clearly noticeable that you can begin to use planned, deliberate increases. Even then it is best to try to increase at a very slow speed to avoid relapses. If, for example, you are getting better by the week, you can increase deliberately once a month. That way you make sure you always keep your surplus. Chapter 7 is about increasing in a safe way and about when it is safe to increase. The advice in that chapter is also applicable to people with severe ME, so I will not discuss it here.

There is, though, one aspect that must be mentioned. When you have been away from activities for a long time, it is not always easy to know what it might be realistic to try out when you are well enough to start reintroducing activities. It is often possible to work out what is realistic by analysing each activity. To watch TV, for example, you must be able to tolerate both movement within your field of vision, light and sound all at once. If you cannot cope with an assistant talking while they are walking about the room, it is not likely that you will be able to watch much TV. In that case you might instead choose activities that are only about either listening or looking, such as thumbing through a catalogue, or listening to music or an audio book.

In the same way a wheelchair ride requires that you can cope with vibrations and sitting up. If the ride is to be outdoors, you must be able to get dressed and leave the house. If that is not possible, you can split this activity up, too. You can get accustomed to sitting in a wheelchair indoors before attempting a trip outside.

When a long time has passed since you last did something, the activity will always need a certain amount of getting used to, even if you really are well enough to do the activity. Do not get surprised if the activities are more tiring than you thought.

Start very carefully, and increase as you feel is natural. In the increasing phase it is important to remember that the main goal is to retain your improvement. To do this you must give higher priority to rest than to activity and make sure to retain your surplus energy at all times, so that the symptom level continues to fall. Otherwise the dramatic symptoms may return. Even when improvement is well-established and you have been able to increase your activity level somewhat, you may find that there is an advantage to having periods of doing a little less in order to bring the symptom level further down. It is very frustrating to reduce the activity level even a little, but you can often notice a positive effect in quite a short time.

COMMUNICATION WITH PROFESSIONALS

Home visits from doctors and other professionals can be paced by adding frequent pauses to the conversation. This may not always be enough. You can save a lot of energy by dictating or writing down key words or sentences ahead of time. When the person arrives you can hand them the page or Dictaphone so they can read, or listen to, it in another room. Afterwards they can come back and ask any supplementary questions. It is even possible to ask for their questions ahead of time, so that you can formulate your answers in a considerably less demanding way. In my experience it is necessary to explain to the professional ahead of time how the visit will be arranged. This can be done by a family member or assistant so that you do not have to use your energy for that.

WHEN HEALTH CARE PROFESSIONALS ARE IMPATIENT

Some people with severe ME find that the health care professionals around them begin to get impatient and attempt to pressurise them to do more and more. When you are very ill, having to educate professionals is the last thing you need. Still, there is much to gain from good communication. First of all it is useful to make a list of examples which explain how ill you actually are, so that people understand that it is not just a question of being very tired. Be concrete. For example, you could explain that you cannot always manage to drink even when you are very thirsty. You do not have to focus solely on the most extreme things; you could use some examples from daily life, too. Examples like those are often quite shocking to the people who hear them. For example, a person from the social services was very shocked when a patient told her that she could go for a walk around the building she lived in, but that if she attempted to walk around the block it would take her two weeks to get over it. The patient did not think of this as extreme at all, but the lady from the social services saw it differently.

It may also be helpful to do what I have mentioned earlier in this chapter – to make a list of any small signs of improvement as they occur. That makes it easier to avoid the professionals getting panicky because they do not think things are improving. It can also be a good idea to explain a little about why you choose to do the things you do. If you say: "No, I am not ready to increase yet," it could be misunderstood as you being afraid to do more. Instead, you can say: "I want to use my new energy on drinking every time I am thirsty." Such an explanation shows that you are having to prioritise drastically but that you do want to do things. This type of communication increases people's understanding of your situation and prevents misinterpretations.

DO NOT GIVE UP HOPE OF GETTING BETTER

A British survey among 2,760 patients showed that 88% of those with ME had been severely ill at one time or another during their illness. When they filled out the questionnaire, 33% of the patients were severely ill, but only 4% were bed-bound. A large number of the patients had, in other words, become better. Research done by the occupational therapist Irma Pinxterhuis has also shown that it is possible to experience improvement in severe ME, even if you have been ill for years. Having severe ME is not necessarily a life sentence. Yet it can sometimes take a long time to see improvement. That does not mean that you will not be much better in the end. In *Cheers* magazine, number 72, Bryony P. says:

> *"I'm 19 now and became ill when I was 13, spending the first few years as a SAM (severely affected member). I'm feeling quite well at the moment, studying with the Open University and even taking dancing and trapeze lessons!"*

Bryony is not the only one who has become much better, so you must not give up hope of becoming one of them.

The most important thing for people with severe ME is the struggle to get enough healing rest, and when you are finally able to increase a little, it must be done with great caution to avoid losing what you have gained.

TASKS

1 Reduce activities as much as possible so symptom flaring is reduced and the amount of healing rest increases.

2 Learn one or more relaxation techniques and use them daily if you can tolerate them.

3 Find some small, pleasant activities that can be done without making you worse. That way you have something to enjoy while waiting to get better.

4 Write down some examples of how much your functional ability is reduced, so they can be given to health care professionals as needed.

5 When the first signs of improvement occur, make sure you make a record of them with the date.

SUMMARY OF CHAPTER 19

1. ME can make social activities difficult, but there are many adjustments that can make it possible to have a satisfying social life.

2. If you want people to understand your limitations they need an explanation. Simple explanations usually work best.

3. Social activities that you take part in on your own are the easiest to adjust to one's own limitations. These include SMS, MMS, online forums and letters. It is also possible to put a limit on the length of telephone calls and visits. This should be agreed on ahead of time.

4. Visiting others can be paced by just taking part for short sessions or by having a rest in another room at some point.

5. Other activities outside the home can be adapted to your needs with energy saving aids, rest breaks and the like.

CHAPTER 19:

SOCIAL ACTIVITIES

INTRODUCTION

Pacing of social activities is especially challenging. When you are alone, you can do things the way that is best suited to your needs, and you can easily change your plans along the way as needed. When you are with others, you have to consider their wishes, needs and expectations too. The result can easily end in you doing too much. In this chapter I describe how you can set up social activities so that the strain will not become too great and how you can communicate with others so that they understand why the social gathering has to be set up in a certain way.

COMMUNICATION

In order to understand why you need adjustments in social connections, it is important to explain things properly to people. If you attempt to hide that you are ill or you make your arrangements without saying anything, there is a greater risk of hitting misunderstandings or even scepticism. This explanation usually works:

> *"ME is an illness that leads to reduced energy production in the cells. That means that I get drained of energy far more quickly than others, and it takes a long time before I regain strength again afterwards. Therefore it is important that I split everything into small sessions which don't use up all my energy, and that I take frequent rest breaks. This is called pacing and is one of the most recommended treatments internationally. I don't enjoy it but it is better than getting more and more ill because I do too much all the time. You can help me keep my health as good as possible by helping me stop in time."*

Saying that people can help you is important because it makes people feel useful instead of rejected. It is also important to include the information about pacing being a treatment that is recommended internationally. When you follow a treatment that is recommended by your doctor it is easier to get understanding from people than if they think this is something you have thought up yourself. It is usually enough to use a short explanation for acquaintances, but closer family and friends may wish to know more. In that case you can let them read Chapter 1 of this book. It may also be useful to encourage them to read a leaflet or booklet on ME. Many national ME associations have good ones you can use. For instance, the leaflet *Quick Tour of ME*, published by The Young ME Sufferers Trust, which is available on www.thymestrust.org.

Good communication does not solve all problems, but it helps avoid unnecessary misunderstandings. Just as the people with ME need time to accept that they are ill, the people around them do too. The feelings others go through are much the same, but everyone goes through them at different speeds. This can be a challenge for all parties concerned. Not everyone faces the reality that someone they know well has a chronic illness. This, of course, is disappointing. When things are at their worst it can help to remember that some people come back strongly when they have adjusted to the situation.

LONG-DISTANCE COMMUNICATION

The social activities that are the easiest to adapt are those that you do alone, like sending text messages, writing messages or letters, or taking part in an online forum. These activities can be done in small sessions and you can answer when it suits you. You can read more about this in the paragraph on 'Reading, Writing and Communication' in Chapter 23, 'Tips for Energy Conservation'.

If you would like a bit of a change, virtual vacations (pretend trips) and long-distance parties are a way to create variation. Both of these are mainly about imagination, but you can add extra activities at will. You can look at pictures from your chosen destination, eat a meal from the area, listen to or read about where you are planning to go, etc. You can adapt how much you take part and for how long. Any extra activities can be spread over several days. It is particularly nice if you can get some friends who could join you long-distance. You get a feeling of belonging just by knowing that others are doing the same thing you are, but it is even more fun if you are well enough to communicate via SMS or internet. Online groups like Facebook are well suited for these sort of long-distance arrangements.

An example of an invitation to this sort of event can be found in Worksheet 10. At the time of publication, a range of free virtual experiences can be downloaded from www.clairewade.com. These are created specifically for people with ME, and have pictures, text and audio material, plus a range of suggestions for supplementary activities.

One disadvantage about long-distance communication is that not everyone is good at answering emails and text messages. People would often like to take part, but it ends up getting lost in the rush of busy days. Sometimes it is easier to keep regular contact with people who are prepared for a long-distance friendship from the start. People you met often before are not always capable of adapting to keeping up the contact in other ways.

TELEPHONE CONVERSATIONS

Telephone conversations are a good way to stay in contact with the rest of the world when you cannot be out much, but it is very easy to end up talking for far too long. It is worth deciding ahead of time how long you want the call to last and to set an alarm that can let you know when the time is up. It also helps to warn the other person that the conversation will be short. Saying something like: *"I can only manage to talk for five minutes, but I did so want to talk to you anyway"*, is a nice message, which people do not take as a rejection. You can also ask people to help you stop when the alarm goes off. It can be a smart idea to set the alarm to ring a minute or two before the limit so that you have time to wind up the conversation. Short, frequent phone calls are better than fewer, longer ones.

Not everyone is easy to get hold of on the phone and it can be tiring to have to call again and again. You can save some energy by sending a text message to agree on a time for the call that suits both. An answering machine is a good idea when it does not suit to answer calls. You can also turn your mobile phone off or put it on silent. Sometimes you have to ask people to call back later. Zoë Williams suggests the following wording in her collection of tips for people with ME:

> *"I'm sorry, but I am not well enough to talk just now. Can we arrange a time when I can call you back?"*

Phone calls from telephone salespeople and charities raising funds take far too much energy. *There may be a register in your country which you can join to reduce the number of unsolicited marketing calls you receive.* In some countries there are separate registers for telephone sales and charity phone calls. You may have to join these registers individually. *Going ex-directory may also reduce the number of unwanted calls.*

VISITS

When it comes to visits it is a must to plan the length of the visit ahead of time. When you have not seen people much for a long time, it is very easy to end up talking until you collapse. Therefore, it is important to explain to your guest ahead of time how long the visit will last. Ideally, it is good to use an alarm to remind you of when it is time to stop. If other family members take part in the visit it can be useful to ask them to help with stopping the visit in time. It is perfectly possible to take rest breaks during a visit. This is especially simple if other family members can talk to the person while you are resting. If you live alone, you can offer the guest a newspaper or something else that will not disturb you while you are resting.

If you would like to serve something to eat or drink, you can choose something that takes a minimum of preparation, like fruit, potato chips/crisps, or bought cookies. Tea or coffee can be prepared ahead of time and served in a thermos so you do not wear yourself out rushing around making coffee just as the guests arrive. Or you could set up your kitchen with labels so it's easier for guests to make themselves a drink. If you find it tiring to talk, but can manage to do other things, it is possible to invite people to, for example, listen to music, watch TV or take part in a hobby. You must not think that people will not be bothered to come just because you cannot talk all the time.

A young Norwegian man called Øistein has a big brother with severe ME who can only whisper a few words at a time. He cannot tolerate other people talking much either. Øistein visits him anyway. *"When I am there I potter around and do the things the assistants haven't the time for. It's really about being with him, because that is what I want. Be there for him."* Visiting someone who cannot talk much (or not at all) is not something that only brothers do. Zoë Williams is in her thirties and has been bed-bound for many years. In her experience, inviting people to just come and be with her has worked well. Her friends do Sudoku, read or do other things that do not make a lot of noise while she rests. Visits like that can lessen the feeling of being cut off and alone in the world. Zoë says:

> *"Sometimes having a guest who is understanding and adaptable enough to visit without talking a lot, makes the difference between being totally isolated and being able to have some quiet company."*

If you are severely or very severely ill and need suggestions as to what you can do with friends and family, you can read *Bed without Boundaries* by the British art therapist Lois G. Owen. The book is in the bibliography.

VISITING OTHERS

If you are able to visit others, the same principles for making necessary adaptations apply. If you are invited to a family birthday party it can be necessary to arrive late, leave early and take rest breaks while there. You can arrive just before dinner is served and just stay for the dinner, or you can just come for coffee afterwards. Family members might like to stay at the party longer, but you may need to go home early. This can be difficult if you are dependent upon the family members for transportation. In that case you can check whether there is a room with a bed that you can borrow so that you can rest. That way you can stay longer without getting worn out. It is a good idea to bring ear defenders and ear plugs with you so the noise from the guests does not become a problem. You can also use these while you are with the others. Remember that there may be other energy conservation measures you can do to your advantage, like sitting with your legs up, or bringing a bean bag to sit/lie on.

TRIPS OUT OF THE HOUSE

Shopping, cinema and café trips are activities that do not have to be social since you can do them alone. Yet these are things one often does with others and, in any case, they are quite stimulating. That is why I am bringing them up here. The most important thing to think about is that activities out of the house are far more exhausting than lounging at home. That means that they must be built up gradually, especially if it is a long time since the last time you did them. The best way is to start by doing the activity alone or with someone who functions solely as a chauffeur or assistant. You start by doing something that only takes a few minutes, like a trip to the corner shop or the nearest kiosk. The first times you go to a shop it is not a good idea to go because there is something you need to get, like a birthday present. If you do that you are more likely to stay in the shop far too long. If you would like to buy something, stick to something you know they have, like a magazine or a snack.

Besides making sure the trip is a short one, you should also think about which energy conservation measures you can take. These might be sunglasses, ear defenders, a wheelchair or a camping stool to sit on if you have to wait in line. When you are well enough to be in a shop for 15-20 minutes you can try a trip to a café. It is better to start with a café than a restaurant because it often takes longer before your food is served in a restaurant. When you can manage to cope with a trip to a café that lasts an hour, trying to go to a restaurant is realistic. A trip to the cinema must be built up in a different way because it is difficult to leave in the middle of a film. Instead, you build up watching films at home. When you can manage to watch an entire film at home, and you also can manage the car ride and being pushed in a wheelchair or walk the distance necessary to get into the cinema, you are ready to try a trip there. Remember to check beforehand how long the film lasts.

When you have taken a few trips and know more or less what you can handle, it is time to think about inviting a friend along. It is smart to start with only one person, and preferably someone who is prepared to do things on your terms. You can always invite more people later. It is more demanding to be with several people at a time, so you may have to cut down on the time you can spend with them compared to what you can manage when you are alone. This can be done by turning up a bit later than the others. Since it is often no fun to have to leave before the others, it can be easier to come late and leave at the same time the others do. You can also put in a bit of rest along the way by, for example, dropping one shop on a shopping trip and resting instead in a corner on your own. Another method is to rest on a chair in a fitting room, or even by going to a toilet and sitting quietly for a while on the seat. If you have a wheelchair with you, you can rest every time you find a quiet space.

Public buildings, like airports, train stations and shopping centres usually have a rest room, often in connection with the toilets. A classic trick is to rest on a mattress in a furniture shop, or a sofa at a café, and, of course, you can rest in the car before going home or between errands. The most creative idea I have come across is lying down to rest in a solarium that is not turned on. This only works if the solarium is close to where you are going. With a mixture of creativity, courage and the will-power to put in place the necessary adjustments, you will often be able to feel that you are enjoying yourself as much as the others, even if you do have to do things a bit differently. It is, however, absolutely necessary that you start step by step and very carefully by first increasing the activities when you are well enough to do it without getting a symptom increase. Otherwise your nice trip will assuredly end up leading straight to symptom increases and maybe even a relapse.

****

Many people with ME have periods when they wish for more social life than they can manage. But there are ways to find adjustments that make it possible to have a degree of contact with the rest of the world. As your health improves you will find that you can gradually resume the social activities that had to be set aside for a period. You are not condemned to a lonely life.

TASKS

1 Consider which social activities are suitable for you right now and which adjustments you will need.

2 Take the initiative for social activities as often as you can manage. Try to do it regularly, for example once a week or once a month.

3 Think about how you will explain your adjustments to your guest/s. The explanation can be written down or dictated and given to the guests. If anyone else is doing the explaining for you, it is a good idea to figure out what you want them to say and not say.

SUMMARY OF CHAPTER 20

1. It is a challenge to take part in big events like weddings and confirmations if one is not able to take part the same way as everyone else.

2. There are a large number of possible adjustments and solutions, both for those who have to stay at home and for those who can join some parts of an event.

3. It is easier making adjustments to an event if you start planning a good while ahead of time.

4. If the big event is your own, you can arrange it exactly the way you want and need. Think unconventionally. If the event is someone else's you do not have quite as much freedom, but there are still a number of adjustments that can be made.

5. If you have to stay at home you could perhaps watch some of the event via video transmission on your phone (e.g. Skype, or recorded videos), or use some of the other suggestions in this chapter.

6. If you can take part, you can use energy-saving techniques, such as having a camp bed in a back room so you can rest.

CHAPTER 20:

BIG EVENTS

INTRODUCTION

Big events can be a challenge if you are not well enough to take part in the same way as others. Yet there are a number of adjustments that can make it possible to take part in or mark the event your own way.

ATTITUDE

When you cannot take part in an event the normal way, it is a challenge emotionally. Grief reactions are not unusual. It can be an advantage to cry or rant and rage before you start planning how to make adjustments, because it is easier to be constructive when you have cooled down emotionally. When you get as far as doing the actual planning, it helps if you can work up a bit of enthusiasm. If you are thinking you now have to figure out a poor substitute for what you should have been able to enjoy, there is, unfortunately, a risk that the event you plan will actually be a poor substitute. If, on the other hand, you can manage to think: *"Now I am going to arrange a really great party on my own terms, and within my limits"*, there is a good chance that the event will be really nice for you.

PREPARATIONS

When you are planning adjusted events you should start far ahead of time. Often you can get the most out of things by thinking unconventionally and doing your own thing. It is a good idea to do a lot of the planning yourself instead of waiting for others to make some kind of arrangement. Not all healthy people are good at seeing opportunities instead of hindrances.

Before you begin to plan your event it is a good idea to know where you stand. These questions may be useful to consider:

1. How ill am I?

2. Which activities can I handle, and in how large doses?

3. If I wish to do more than usual, how much can I do without getting a big relapse?

4. Which parts of the event can others help me with, and which do I need to do myself?

5. What financial resources do I have available?

Remember that you will have less energy for the event itself if you have to do a lot of the preparations yourself. It can be handy to keep this in mind. In addition, it is a good idea to think about the fact that most people with ME have a tendency to overestimate how much they can do. Some people with ME say that when they plan a vacation, they make a list of all the sights they want to see. Then they read the list again and remove half of the items. A while later, they reconsider the list and remove another half. Then they are left with a programme they can manage to get through. It is not always necessary to be this drastic every time, but if you are going to do something you have not done for a long time you have to keep in mind that it will be far more tiring than you are used to. I once read about a young woman with quite severe ME who went on her honeymoon straight after the wedding. The result was that she was bed-bound for a period afterwards because of overexertion. It is this kind of relapse you can often avoid with realistic planning and creative solutions. Below you will find a long list of suggestions for solutions people with ME have enjoyed. Choose what you like and let yourself be inspired.

YOUR OWN EVENTS

When the big event is your own you have many opportunities to adjust things. One of the most common adjustments is to split up the event, so that the ceremony and the party are on separate days. You can also have several smaller parties instead of one big one. Be aware that ceremonies like weddings and confirmations can be held at home. Sometimes a long-distance party is more suitable than the usual kind. You can read more about long-distance parties in the sections on 'Long-Distance Communication' in Chapter 19, 'Social Activities'. Basically you can choose any size and form of event that suits you and your health. When the event is a family affair, too, it should usually be possible to arrange the programme in a way that includes the family member who is ill.

If you need ideas on how to arrange a party there are books and web pages with ideas that you can adapt. An example of such a website is: http://stylecaster.com/101-theme-party-ideas/

WHEN YOU ARE TOO ILL TO TAKE PART

There are a number of ways to adapt events even if you are unable to join in in the usual way. Sometimes you can have the party at home, or in the garden, so that you can spend a short time with the guests or see the party from the window. Even if you cannot manage to go out and join the guests some of them can come and say hello or chat. At other times it will be more suitable for the person whose event it is to drop in for a short visit, either on the big day or at another time. That way you get to give them a gift personally. You could also ask that official photos are taken where you live so that you too can be in the photos.

Sometimes you can eat the same food that the other guests are having and have the same table decorations, even if you must stay at home. Alternatively, people can come by the next day with something nice from the event for you to eat. If you have a phone that can go online, somebody who is there can call and hold their phone so that you can glimpse the event via a video-call, or maybe even talk to people. You could also be kept up-to-date using MMS and SMS. Sometimes it is possible to see the party by web camera. A classic solution is to see the event on video afterwards. Many events are videoed anyway.

It is easier to feel included if you have a precise timetable so that you know what is happening when. That way you can take part by listening to the same music, eating the same dessert when they are having theirs, etc. If you would like to give a speech, you can have it videotaped ahead of time and shown during the party, or write it down and have it read by someone else if that is easier.

You can make your own parallel ceremony. You can light some candles, listen to music, send a helium balloon out of the window or anything else you feel will match the mood and give a sense of marking the event. This is often the best solution for funerals, where many of the other suggestions are unsuitable.

IF YOU CAN JOIN THE EVENT

When those arranging the event are not close family you will have far less influence on the arrangements. Yet there are still alternatives. In *AYME Graduates Newsletter*, 13th of August, 2005, Diane S. wrote about the time when she was asked to be a close friend's bridesmaid. At the time Diane was still so ill that she seldom left the house. It was therefore necessary to make a number of adaptations. The first thing she did was to book a room at the hotel where the wedding celebrations were to be held. That way she could rest during the party and stay the night afterwards. She also arranged with a mutual friend that she would function as her assistant during the party. During the ceremony, Diane used a wheelchair in order to save energy, and the friend pushed the chair. Afterwards she rested in her room until the party started and during large parts of it. Her friend kept her up-to-date by text, and came in to take her out in the wheelchair every time something special was about to happen, like cutting the cake. Afterwards, Diane summed it up:

> *"...With the right planning and determination... it really is possible to enjoy a special event without feeling like we are missing out."*

When you join in on big events you usually want to stay as long as possible. You should consider using energy conservation techniques you do not usually need. Ear defenders/ear plugs and a wheelchair can make it possible for someone who is usually able to walk around to last for a longer time. At other times you might need a camp bed in a back room so you can rest, or a garden chair that can be reclined so you can sit comfortably. It is also a good idea to have a chat with the host concerning whether there are important parts of the programme that you particularly want to experience, or that they wish you to take part in. That way you can take the rest breaks you need in between without missing the best bits.

Another important thing is to do all preparations as far ahead of time as possible. Clothes, gifts, etc. should be bought a long time before the event so that you can get as much rest as possible. Some preparations that most people would do the same day can be done ahead of time. You can pack your bags several days ahead of time and shower the day before, so that the only thing you have to do on the day itself is eat, dress and put on make-up if you want to.

In connection with big events people often feel that it is worth feeling poorly for a while afterwards. But you do not want to end with a long-lasting relapse. In Chapter 5 there is a recipe for planning overexertions without ending up with lasting consequences. If you plan things the right way you can often take part in big events one way or another. If you are lucky you can say, like Diane, that you did not feel that you missed out on anything.

TASKS

1 When you are planning a big event start by evaluating your situation. You can use these questions:

- How ill am I?

- Which activities can I manage and for how long?

- If I would like to do more than usual, how much can I arrange without getting a big relapse?

- Which parts of the event can others help with and which must I do myself?

- What financial resources are available?

2 Find out whether there are parts of the event that you can manage to get to, if desired, and which adjustments you need?

3 Are there possible alternatives for the things you cannot join in with? Try to be creative and think outside the box.

SUMMARY OF CHAPTER 21

1. Research shows that people with ME have a number of disturbances in physical functioning that make it impossible to exercise normally.

2. In the unstable stage exercise will lead to relapse, no matter whether you are mildly, moderately or severely ill. In the stabilising stage people with moderate and mild ME can have tiny doses of movement as part of a varied range of activities. In the improvement stage everybody can tolerate some physical activity/exercise, but people with severe ME often find that activities of daily living provide as much movement as they can handle.

3. In order to avoid movement being damaging, you must split it into very small sessions that do not lead to symptom increase. Just one or two movements during the day can be as much as a person with ME can physically tolerate.

4. The forms of movement that are suitable for people with ME are types where you use gentle, slow movements and it can be good to combine movements with relaxation exercises.

5. ME cannot be exercised away. What can help with ME are pacing, rest and certain medical treatments, not exercise.

CHAPTER 21:

PACING OF MOVEMENT

INTRODUCTION

Like all other activities, movement can be paced. However, not everyone with ME is well enough to do movements, and by no means all forms of movement are suitable for people with ME. This chapter is about when it is possible to do gentle exercise and how it can be done so that it does not lead to relapse.

When you say the word exercise, most people think of jogging, weightlifting, aerobics and other forms of training that are normal among healthy people. These forms of exercise are usually far too strenuous for ME patients to safely manage, even when done in tiny sessions. The idea that exercise is good for everyone is a common misunderstanding. Forget everything about exercising ME away – it simply cannot be done. It is, however, very easy to exercise your way into a relapse. So focus on learning pacing. Introduce movement only when it feels natural and your body is able to tolerate it.

I have chosen to use the word 'movement' in this chapter to avoid the misunderstandings that can occur by using the word 'exercise'. In some places I use the word 'exercises' to indicate deliberate movements separate from activities of daily living.

If you have an illness or an injury you should, of course, take this into consideration when moving. Individual limits vary among healthy people, and vary even more among people with ME. For people with severe ME, being turned over in bed in conjunction with care can be as much movement as their body can tolerate, while this would be far too little for someone who is not bed-bound. The variation is not just about how much your body can cope with, but also about which stage you are at. In some stages the illness is so acute that exercises cannot be done safely, while suitably adjusted exercises may be possible in other stages. We will look more closely at this.

WHY PEOPLE WITH ME CANNOT EXERCISE NORMALLY

There are disturbances of physical functioning in ME that explain why patients cannot exercise normally. One of these is the lack of ability to produce enough energy in the cells. This has been shown in a number of research papers. The findings are numerous and complicated. Because of that there is not room to go into detailed explanations here. Some of this is explained in more detail in Chapter 22, 'Background and Discussion'. Readers who would like to know more can read the article, *The Physiology of Exercise Intolerance in Patients with Myalgic Encephalomyelitis (ME) and the Utility of Graded Exercise Therapy* by S. Pierce and P.W. Pierce. A broader discussion can be found in *Myalgic Encephalomyelitis – Adult and Paediatric: International Consensus Primer for Medical Practitioners* by Bruce Carruthers et al.

The research is clear: exhaustion in ME has a physical explanation. You do not feel tired or exhausted because you have done too little and become deconditioned – there is a pathological mechanism that leads to actual energy deficiency. Physical movement cannot cure the basic illness. ME cannot be exercised away and it is not possible to reach a normal level of functioning by exercising.

People with ME are injured by training, which healthy people handle with no problems. The following is an example: *"My consultant told me to take at least an hour of hard physical exercise every day. I followed the exercise programme for a few weeks. I was, at first, physically sick and very soon became unable to do anything other than the one hour of exercise. Finally, I was unable to do even that and needed many weeks in bed to get over it. I returned to the doctor unable to walk at all."* (20-year old with ME.) This quote, which appears in *Somebody help ME* by Jill Moss, illustrates how bad things can get when people with ME exercise in the wrong way. It has become fairly well known that people with ME cannot exercise in the same way healthy people can. What is not so well known is that people with ME get can get some benefit (but not illness improvement) from tiny doses of exercise which are too small to make any difference in a healthy person. The opportunity to utilise this is one of the themes in this chapter.

VERY RESTRICTED LIMITS

When the Danish physiotherapist Manette Garde started treating ME patients, she was shocked by how little it took before the movement was too much, but also by how big a change it was possible to get with really minimal doses of movement. To illustrate this she said that she had a patient who was moderately ill, but not among the healthiest in this group. Garde prepared a movement programme made up of a series of movements, but the patient was told to only do one of each movement. The programme was carried out once a fortnight and led to a great change in flexibility and strength.

The change was much greater than expected based on the amount of movement. When Garde suggested that the patient could do each movement twice, this small increase led to a two-week relapse. Garde found it frightening that there was such a small difference between a programme with a good effect and a programme that made things worse. This example is by no means unique. Actually, the limits of severely affected patients are even more restricted. It is vital that patients and health care professionals are knowledgeable about how little an ME patient can tolerate. Pacing, rest and some medical treatments, among others treating infections and immune modulating treatments, can lead to improvement in people with ME. This can give a clear improvement in the level of functioning and make an increased amount of movement possible.

WHICH ME PATIENTS CAN DO EXERCISES?

It is easy to assume that people with mild ME can do exercises while people with severe ME cannot. It is, unfortunately, not that simple. Whether movements are possible or not depends more on the stage you are at than on how ill you are. In Chapter 11, Dr. Franklin's three stages of illness activity are described. The stages are very useful for judging whether movements are possible.

In the unstable stage both the symptoms and the activity level vary greatly and the patient has an overall high symptom level. In this stage attempts at movements usually lead to relapse no matter the level of functioning. Therefore, stabilising the illness process and reducing the symptom level are important for people in the unstable stage. Movements can and must wait until later.

The stabilising stage is characterised by greater stability and the symptoms calming down. At this stage people with moderate and mild ME can have tiny doses of movements as part of a varied activity menu. People with severe ME cannot usually do movements at this stage. Daily activities, like moving a little in bed or changing clothes, are usually enough movement for them. It is not until towards the very end of the stabilising stage that you can gradually increase movements without having to pay for it by cutting down on other activities.

The improvement stage is distinguished by the improvement developing so quickly that you can increase activities frequently. At this stage everyone can do some movements, dependent upon one's physical level of functioning. Many people with severe ME will find that daily activities like sitting up for a bit or walking to the toilet etc., are as much movement as they can tolerate. People with ME, at all levels, are fully capable of evaluating which activities and what degree of movement is realistic, and must never be pressured to do anything other than (or more than) they themselves find appropriate. In the improvement stage you can increase your movements at the same rate you increase other activities. But you must not even think of only increasing movement. Unbalanced activities increase the danger of relapse. This is especially true for physical activities, but also for all other activities. It is far better for your body to have varied and adaptable activities. If you are unsure of which stage you are at you can read more about them in Chapter 11, 'Three Stages – Three Management Strategies'. Usually one is at one of the first two stages. There are not normally very many people at the improvement stage.

HOW DO YOU PLAN FOR EXERCISE?

In order to avoid relapse it is absolutely necessary to plan movement correctly. On a good day it is easy to fall for the temptation to keep on doing the exercises, but this MUST be avoided. Healthy people, too, have a tendency to push too hard, but they only get stiff the next day. People with ME risk serious, long-lasting relapses. You must therefore, ahead of time and carefully, plan how long a spell should last and make sure that it is suited to your level of functioning. Activities that you are not used to are generally more tiring than things you are used to, so it is important to start out very carefully.

There are several rules of thumb to help you. The first is that little and often is a better strategy than doing larger doses occasionally. One spell of five minutes per day will be far less tiring than half an hour once a week. The second rule of thumb is to split up the exercise spells. You could for example do five single movements at different times of the day instead of doing all five in a row. People who can do a bit more could split up a fifteen-minute spell into three five-minute spells. This way of thinking is like interval training, but for people with ME the spells must be very short. Many will also need more time to rest between spells than is normal in interval training. People with ME also often need more than the usual amount of variation.

Variation is the third rule of thumb. Repetition is not good for people with ME. It is better for your body to do five totally different movements than to do the same movement five times. You can have short spells with different forms of movements instead of doing the same type all the time. Instead of just walking, or bending and stretching, you can set up a combination that is tailored to your needs. When you plan variation it is a good idea to take into consideration the movements you are already doing in your daily life. You can plan movements that involve other parts of the body and other muscles than those you usually use. An example could be that if you already walk up and down lots of stairs at home you are not likely to benefit from practising movements that are similar to walking up and down stairs.

The fourth and most important rule is that movement must remain within your limits. This means that you must not feel particularly tired afterwards, and that you must not experience pain. In ME, pain is a sign that you have kept on for far too long. A movement session must be so short that your body feels comfortably used. After resting for as long as you usually rest you should feel so well that you can continue with your usual activities. You are not supposed to be wiped out all day after a session of movements. This usually means the sessions must be quite short. Few people with moderate ME can manage more than five to ten minutes, and in the beginning you should usually start with far shorter sessions. One of the biggest challenges with such short spells is remembering to do them. The easiest way to remember is to do the movements at a particular time of day, or to connect the movements to other activities, for example doing two single movements in connection with heading towards the toilet. This option should not be chosen if getting to the toilet is tiring in itself, of course.

In short, the principles for pacing movement are exactly the same as for pacing other activities. With other activities, what works are small, varied doses carried out within one's limits. This goes for movement, too.

PROGRESSIVE MUSCLE RELAXATION AS MOVEMENT

Progressive muscle relaxation is a form of relaxation technique that switches between tightening and relaxing certain muscles in the body. In healthy people this gives deep relaxation. This technique tires people with ME. For them it does not lead to relaxation – instead it gives the same effect as exercise. Progressive muscle relaxation is therefore not well suited as relaxation for people with ME. Instead, you can content yourself with just feeling the different areas of your body. Since people with ME often get exercise effect from single movements, progressive muscle relaxation can be used as a very gentle exercise programme (for those who can tolerate it). When the functional ability of people with severe ME begins to improve, tightening and relaxing muscles when lying flat can be the only form of exercise that is possible. Even so, such movements must be done with great caution, and not until the improvement process is well established.

For people with moderate and mild ME it can be useful to start off very carefully as a transition to something more active later. You might use relaxation CDs with instructions in progressive muscle relaxation to learn the technique. In the beginning you only listen to the instructions, even if you are mildly ill and think that you will manage the movements with no problems. After a while you can slowly increase the number of movements. You start with one movement only and increase gradually. One of the disadvantages of instructions from a CD is that the instructor goes through the movements in a certain order: First you tighten the muscles in your feet, then the legs, the knees, etc. This is considerably more tiring than splitting the movements into groups that use different body parts. You could, for example, do a movement with your legs, then with your arms and then with your body or head. It is also easier to do several small groups like this a day than to do the whole programme at once.

The CD *Energise and Relax with Yoga* by Angela Stevens is a useful starting point. Diana Lampen also has several similar sessions. Please see the list 'Pathfinder to movement for people with ME' at the back of the book. A physiotherapist who is knowledgeable about ME can set up a programme for the individual patient.

WHICH OTHER TYPES OF MOVEMENT ARE SUITABLE FOR PEOPLE WITH ME?

When you are well enough to do more than single movements, there are several different forms you could try out. A type of movement that can be suitable for people with ME is one that uses slow, gentle movements and which often combines the movements with relaxation. The most popular movement systems among people with ME are gentle yoga, qigong, the Alexander Technique, Basic Body Awareness Therapy and walking. There are no comparative studies that show which of these forms of exercise are best. The important thing is to find out which form of movement your body finds most suitable and which can be done within your body's own limits. As long as these requirements are fulfilled it probably makes no difference which technique you choose. All of these can be done at home or through a course. Exercising at home is usually the most suitable for most people with ME since one can do things at one's own speed and do not have to go anywhere. A list of books, CDs and DVDs with instructions for home use can be found at the back of the book. Another way of moving is to do stretching exercises, but here, too, you must be very careful, since stretching exercises often lead to using several muscle groups at once. This is too strenuous for many people with ME.

Walking is most probably the commonest form of movement among people who are not bed-bound. Going for walks is suitable for people who can walk freely indoors and who have enough surplus energy to manage to walk without losing any of their indoor walking distance. Walking needs no instruction, few preparations and, on top of this, it is free of charge. Another advantage is that walking strengthens the skeleton – it means the bones carry the weight of the body, which helps to prevent osteoporosis by increasing bone density. The biggest problem with walking is calculating the walk so that you can manage to walk home again. This can be done by planning the walk ahead of time or by setting an alarm. If you can walk for five minutes, you set the alarm to ring after two and a half minutes, so you know when it is time to turn back. As with all movement in ME, walking must take place within your body's limits. You should feel comfortable both while walking and afterwards. This may mean just walking to and from the garden gate. When your functional ability improves, you can increase in a controlled way, such as the one described in Chapter 7, 'Improvement and Increasing Activity'.

GROUP TRAINING

Group training is only suitable for people with ME if the illness is mild or moderate, even if it is adapted for people with ME. You should only try group sessions if the trip to and from the place where the exercises are done is not a problem. Those who feel tired from the trip will find that the movements themselves are too exhausting. Be aware that you cannot be sure that you can manage as much as the others even though the course is meant for ME patients. Think ahead – how much should you do? You could, for example, decide to try just one or two of each movement the first time, until you know the programme and have an idea of how much you can manage. Talk to the instructor about this ahead of time so you do not get criticized for not trying hard enough. For most people with ME it is easier to attend a group once a week than to take part in an intensive weekend course. You should not take part in an intensive weekend course in a form of movement that is new to you. In the chapter called 'Pathfinder to Movement Resources for People with ME' you can find tips on how to find movement groups for people with ME.

In some countries, some rehabilitation centres have courses for people with ME. In Norway, the centres themselves say that their courses are only suitable for people with mild to moderate ME. I have read about the experiences of numerous ME patients who have stayed at rehabilitation centres in Norway. Their experiences suggest that it is the healthiest patients who are least likely to relapse as a result of the stay. The more ill the patient is the more likely/certain it is that they will relapse, even if the stay is specially designed for people with ME. General rehabilitation courses are even more likely to cause relapses; staff who are not familiar with ME tend to overestimate patients' levels of health, and pressurise them to do far more than they are capable of doing safely.

In Norway, a minority of rehabilitation centres base their approach on Cognitive Behavioural Therapy and Graded Exercise Therapy. Patients have to be practically recovered to manage these stays without a relapse. You can read more about Cognitive Behavioural Therapy and Graded Exercise Therapy in Chapter 22, 'Background and Discussion'. The Norwegian centres which base their approach on pacing usually have a far gentler programme that is suitable for a larger number of patients. Even so, people need to be relatively well to cope with greater indoor walking distances, eating in a dining room and so on, in addition to the programme itself. If you are considering a stay at a rehabilitation centre, it is vitally important to check their set-up ahead of time to make sure that you are well enough to go through with it. This goes for taking part in other group courses, too. Communicate with other people with ME who have experienced the course, but make sure you ask in great detail both about the stay and their state of health to find out if their situation is at all comparable to yours.

MASSAGE

Massage is one of the quickest ways to increase blood flow to the muscles of healthy people, but not everyone with ME is well enough to be massaged or to be touched at all. When I started physiotherapy I had been gradually improving for several years but was still bed-bound. The first time the physiotherapist gently stroked my legs I was so tired afterwards that I could not walk for an hour. In people who are well enough, massage can loosen tight muscles and lessen pain.

Massage must be given the right way in order to have a positive effect. According to the physiotherapist Merete Sparre, massage for ME should neither be deep, hard nor painful. The code word here, too, is pacing. Massage must be done so gently and in sessions so short that you do not get negative effects afterwards. This may mean that you get a positive effect from two massage grips, while four makes your muscles hard and sore. Not everyone has such narrow limits. Yet it is normal for people with ME to have a much lower tolerance of massage than healthy people have, even when they feel that massage does them good. The rule of thumb for massage is the same as for all other activities: If it feels good and does not give negative effects afterwards, then it is safe to be massaged. If not, you should reduce the amount, or drop the massage.

PHYSIOTHERAPY

Most people connect physiotherapy with exercise. It is less well-known that physiotherapists learn techniques for relaxation and energy conservation as part of their curriculum. This means that physiotherapists can teach these techniques to people with ME. For example, a physiotherapist can watch while you do different activities and give you suggestions as to how these can be done with less effort. They can also teach you relaxation. For people with ME this kind of physiotherapy will be much more useful than pure movement. Learning relaxation and energy conservation is suitable for people in an unstable phase, but for this group it is absolutely necessary for the sessions to be very short and for them to stay within the person's limits. This will often mean that you must take rest breaks during the sessions and that the physiotherapist should make home visits. If you begin to get better, the physiotherapist can tailor a movement programme.

You may want to find out if it is possible to get hold of a physiotherapist with experience of the Basic Body Awareness Therapy (BBAT). BBAT is a form of physiotherapy which uses relaxation and gentle movement to enhance healthy body awareness. Healthy body awareness makes pacing easier. Relaxation improves quality of rest, and the gentle movements used are well suited to people with ME, provided that the sessions are short enough. In some countries, such as the Netherlands, BBAT is a standard technique that is taught to physiotherapists at university. This means that most younger physiotherapists will at least have had an introduction to it. In other countries, such as the UK, the method is virtually unknown.

Physiotherapy has certain disadvantages, though. First of all, physiotherapists usually start off with doing an assessment of the patient's condition. That in itself can lead to the person with ME overdoing it. You should discuss this with the physiotherapist ahead of time and explain the need to split the assessment process up into several visits. If you have written sentences about your activity level, as described in Chapter 1, or have an activity diary, you could show these to the physiotherapist. This leaves the physiotherapist with less work to do on the assessment. In Chapter 18 on severe ME, there is some advice on communication with professionals that can also be used by those who are less ill.

There is another challenge too. A lot of people with ME feel embarrassed about how little they are capable of doing and feel that they ought to be able to do a lot more, or feel under pressure to do more. It is very important to give the physiotherapist as realistic a picture as possible, and to dare to give feedback, even when the exercises or plans do not work. *"The suggestions you made last time haven't worked out very well"*, is important feedback that the physiotherapist needs in order to set up a better plan. If the physiotherapist's plan does not work, then there is something wrong with the plan, not with the patient.

A third challenge with physiotherapy is that there are still a lot of physiotherapists who have little or no experience with ME. This does not need to be a hindrance. It is possible to get some very positive experiences out of co-operating with a physiotherapist who has a friendly and positive approach and is prepared to learn with the patient. Information for health professionals is usually available from patient organisations. Also, in some countries one can find experienced physiotherapists at hospitals or rehabilitation centres who have knowledge of ME and are happy to share it with other physiotherapists. You may even find that some physiotherapists have read this book.

You may experience physiotherapists who are misinformed about ME and think, for example, that graded exercise is suitable for everyone, or that persons with ME have lost the ability to make realistic judgements on how much they are capable of doing. If you want to know why these ideas are incorrect, you can read Chapter 22, 'Background and Discussion'. Unfortunately, there is a great danger that physiotherapists with these sorts of ideas will overestimate how much a person with ME is capable of doing, and will make a plan that will lead to relapse. No one must continue to use a plan that does not work. If information and communication does not improve the co-operation with the physiotherapist, it is better to change physiotherapists. Physiotherapy that involves too much exertion can lead to just as serious a relapse as other forms of overexertion.

WARNING SIGNS

It is important to be on guard when it comes to warning signs that show that it is unsafe to go on with movement. One of the most important things is not to continue with exercises when you have an infection or if you feel like you are coming down with one. Exercise can lead to weakening your immune system and making your infection worse. You can read more about this in the article by Pierce and Pierce, which you can find in the literature list. It is also not a good idea to continue with exercises if you are dealing with extra activities or challenges. A list of situations in which it is not wise to exercise is actually the same as the list of situations when one should not increase the level of activity. This list can be found in Chapter 7, 'Improvement and Increasing Activity'.

One warning sign deserves special mention. The American ME doctor, David Bell, said some years ago that some ME patients experience transitory masking of symptoms in connection with brief, strong physical activity, for example if they run a few metres. The masking is probably caused by endorphins, the body's own painkiller, since hard physical exercise leads to releasing endorphins in healthy people. Releasing endorphins feels good at the time because it makes you feel slightly high, which reduces symptoms. There is, however, a 'hangover' afterwards in the shape of symptom increase due to the overexertion that led to the release of endorphins. Movement in ME should not be so exerting that it leads to endorphins being released, because masking the symptoms makes it very difficult to evaluate how much you can do. Therefore, you usually end up doing too much and have to pay the price afterwards. A much safer way to experience a sensation of well-being is to use relaxation techniques. Relaxation does not lead to side effects for most people with ME. In general, in ME, that which feels good without negative after effects, is safe. This is not true of the high feeling that comes from overexertion.

Masking of symptoms is discussed in more detail in Chapter 12, 'Challenges in Pacing'.

****

Exercise/movement does not produce improvement in ME, and can trigger relapses if you exceed your limits. Two strategies that can increase your chances of improvement are to stabilise your activity at a level that does not give symptoms, and to learn deep rest. When you have managed this and your symptom level is well on its way down, then you can consider adding in movements. Even when you have done all this you must tailor your movements carefully to your symptom level in order to avoid relapse. If your daily activities are varied enough it may well be that you do not need exercises to maintain muscles and flexibility. People with ME do not usually lose much muscle mass, which suggests that they are actually using their body as much as it can tolerate. You can read more about this in Chapter 13, 'Underactivity'. If you should choose to exercise anyway, it is important that you yourself decide the pace. It is pointed out in the Canadian Clinical Treatment Protocol (Carruthers et al.) that *"...externally paced 'Graded Exercise Programmes' or programmes based on the premise that patients are misperceiving their activity limits or illness must be avoided."* Forget anything you have ever heard about exercising away your ME. It is simply not possible. It is, on the other hand, very easy to exercise your way to a relapse. Therefore, focus on learning pacing. Only start with movements when it feels natural and your body is capable of tolerating the exertion.

TASKS

1 Do not start a movement programme until you are stable and improving. If it takes time before you can do any exercises, do not let it make you feel defeated. In any case it is not exercising that makes ME patients better. Focus instead on learning pacing, which can lead to improvement.

2 When you are well enough to do some movements, you must carefully evaluate which forms of movement are suitable for you. Find out which possibilities are available so you have a realistic basis on which to choose.

3 Consider whether you will need help from a physiotherapist or some other professional, or whether you can plan your movements yourself.

4 Investigate how much movement you can safely tolerate. Start at a level that you are sure you can manage without problems. Preferably, you should choose something that seems ridiculously easy. Stick to this level for several weeks. To begin with you should take the amount of time you can safely manage to do activities that are similar to movements, and then start a little lower than that.

5 When you feel it is time to increase the amount of movement, make sure to follow the advice given in Chapter 7, 'Improvement and Increasing Activity'.

SUMMARY OF CHAPTER 22

1. Classic pacing is about getting to know your body's limits, and how to stay within them. The method is based on the fact that ME is a physical illness that leads to an actual reduced capacity for activity.

2. Graded Exercise Therapy (GET) is exercise that is gradually increased, while Cognitive Behaviour Therapy (CBT) is about recognizing and changing negative thought patterns, and increasing the activity level gradually towards a normal level. Both of these treatment methods are based on a theory that chronic fatigue can be due to different triggering events, but are maintained by activity-related anxiety and loss of fitness.

3. The hybrids are made up of different mixtures of pacing, CBT and GET. How the mixtures are put together varies, but usually they put the main focus on gradual increase of activity. The hybrids are a compromise meant to cover all types of chronic fatigue, no matter the cause.

4. The ME patients who have been diagnosed according to fairly strict criteria for diagnosis usually have a long list of physical and biochemical abnormalities that support the theory behind pacing. The abnormalities also explain why these patients get sicker, not just from overexertion and training, but also from gradually increasing activity that is not preceded by improvement. These are strong indications that classic pacing is the management technique that works best for people with strictly defined ME.

5. The theory behind the use of CBT and GET in chronic fatigue may fit some people with chronic fatigue caused by mental illness. However, the theory does not apply to other fatiguing illnesses.

6. The hybrid programmes are suitable for people with physically-caused chronic fatigue who simultaneously suffer from fear of movement, since these programmes take both physical and mental factors into account. On the other hand, the basis for these programmes suggests that the hybrid programmes are not adapted to, and are potentially damaging for, the two other patient groups mentioned in this chapter, that is people with strictly defined ME without additional psychological problems, and people with chronic fatigue as a result of mental illness.

7. Because this book is meant for people with strictly defined ME, I have chosen to present classic pacing, since it is my view that this is the most appropriate management method.

CHAPTER 22:

BACKGROUND AND DISCUSSION

CONFUSION OF TERMS

In order to understand the debate on the management of ME there are two things one must be aware of. One is that the word 'pacing' means different things to different people. Other terms, too, like 'Cognitive Behaviour Therapy' and 'Graded Exercise Therapy', which are discussed later in this chapter, are used differently. We are therefore in a situation where treatment programmes that are called the same thing can be totally different, while programmes that have different names can be almost the same. This makes the situation complicated for patients, researchers and professionals. I have chosen to use the word 'pacing' in this book because it is well-known. I feel that the confusion of terms in this area will only be increased if I chose to use a completely new term at this point.

DIFFERENT CRITERIA DEFINE DIFFERENT PATIENT GROUPS

There are several different sets of criteria for the diagnosis of Chronic Fatigue Syndrome and ME. These different criteria do not define the same group of patients, which further adds to the confusion. Let us therefore take a moment to look at the different diagnostic criteria in use.

The broadest criteria in frequent use are the so-called Oxford criteria. They were published by Michael Sharpe and colleagues in 1991. These are criteria for chronic fatigue as a general phenomenon and not specific criteria for ME or CFS. The Oxford criteria do not exclude patients with depression or anxiety, not even when these conditions alone can explain the patient's illness. In a group of patients diagnosed using the Oxford criteria, therefore, many will suffer from chronic fatigue as a result of mental illness. Others will have fatigue for other reasons, such as undiscovered infections or food intolerances, while it is likely that some have strictly defined neurological ME.

The Fukuda criteria, also called the Centers for Disease Control (CDC) 1994 criteria, are moderately inclusive. They define a considerably more homogeneous patient group than the Oxford criteria, but there are still significant differences between groups of patients. In a study done with Fukuda criteria, one usually finds that a number of patients have approximately the same test results, but that this does not apply to all.

In order to get clearer results many researchers began to use stricter criteria, usually the Canadian Criteria, or the International Consensus Criteria (ICC). Both have Bruce Carruthers as first author, and they were published in 2003 and 2012 respectively. These are criteria for strictly defined neurological ME, which is something very different from broadly defined chronic fatigue.

Because the above-mentioned criteria define different patient groups, research results will vary depending upon which criteria the researchers have chosen. This explains why some research results on Chronic Fatigue Syndrome have been contradictory.

CLASSIC PACING

Patients, carers and professionals have seen that people with ME get strong symptoms as a result of overexertion. This has also been confirmed by a large number of scientific studies. See, among others, Ramsay (1988) and the *International Consensus Criteria (ICC)* by Bruce Carruthers et al (2013), also the *International Consensus Primer for Medical Practitioner*s by the same authors.

Classic pacing aims to prevent symptom flares that follow overexertion by learning to recognize the body's signals. Stopping activities while one still has some energy left provides better conditions for optimizing health. Pacing also stresses switching between activity and rest, choosing undemanding activities and making use of energy-efficient methods of carrying out activities. The goal of classic pacing is to get as much as possible out of the energy one has while at the same time giving the body a chance to recuperate and keep the symptom level at a minimum. Various activity and symptom diaries are often mentioned in books on classic pacing.

Flexible routines are also mentioned, but both are presented as voluntary aids. Most self-help books that were published during the 1980s and 1990s recommend classic pacing. There is a list of these in Figure 1.

Classic pacing is also recommended by the International Association for Chronic Fatigue Syndrome and ME in their primer for physicians, and in the *International Consensus Primer for Medical Practitioners*, both published in 2012. The *Consensus Primer for Medical Practitioners* is written by researchers from the all over the world. The same group are responsible for *The International Consensus Criteria* with Bruce Carruthers as first author.

BOOKS ON CLASSIC PACING

The first self-help book that recommended pacing was published in 1985. It is called *Better Recovery from Viral Illnesses* and is written by the Scottish-Guyanese doctor Darrel Ho-Yen. Ho-Yen's book is still available today, in an updated edition.

CLASSIC PACING IN DIFFERENT COUNTRIES

As with most ME information, much of the writing about pacing comes from Great Britain and the USA. In Britain, classic pacing has been recommended for more than 50 years. The recommendations come from both patient organisations and from researchers, among others Professor Melvin Ramsay. He described the epidemic at the Royal Free Hospital in London in 1955 and continued to do research on ME until he died in 1990. The psychologist Ellen Goudsmit has written several articles on the subject of pacing, most of them patient-oriented. She has also conducted research on the subject. Despite this, only a few controlled research studies were done on pacing in Great Britain. However, there are several studies that have shown good results from this method. Catherine R. Edwards, Andrew Thompson and Alan Blair (2007) did a comprehensive study which showed that people with ME benefit from staying within their limits. Lillebeth Larun and Kirsti Malterud (2007) did a comparative analysis of 20 studies from all over the world. They, too, found that people with CFS benefit from pacing.

FIGURE 1 – BOOKS ON CLASSIC PACING

- William Collinge – *Recovering from ME*, 1993

- Darrel Ho-Yen – *Better Recovery from Viral Illnesses*, 1985 and 1999

- Charles Shepherd – *Living with ME*, 1988 and 1999

- Anne Macintyre – *ME – Post Viral Fatigue Syndrome, How To Live With It*, 1987

- Jill Moss – *Somebody Help ME*, 1995

- Erica Verrillo and Lauren Gellman – *Chronic Fatigue Syndrome – A Treatment Guide,* 1998 and 2012

- Bruce Campbell – *Managing Chronic Fatigue Syndrome and Fibromyalgia*, 2006 and 2010

- Fred Friedberg – *Coping with Chronic Fatigue Syndrome, Nine Things You Can Do*, 1995

See the reference list for more information about the books.

In the United States, William Collinge, a social worker, began organizing management courses based on classic pacing in Incline Village, Nevada, as early as the end of the eighties, after an ME epidemic there. Despite this, the method did not really become generally known in the US before the middle of the nineties and later. This occurred after the psychologist Leonard Jason, and the psychiatrist Fred Friedberg (1997), presented the so-called 'Envelope Theory', which says that if you stay within your limits (i.e. the 'envelope') the symptoms will become milder in time. The symptoms will worsen, though, if you push yourself (i.e. live outside the 'envelope'). Jason and his group of researchers later published several controlled studies of the Envelope Theory, among these one where the physical activity level was measured using an actimeter (a machine which registers movements) carried on the body, while the level of fatigue was measured by questionnaire. The study, which had 44 patients, showed that patients who lived within the 'envelope' had an objective improvement of physical functioning by 37.6% after one and a half years and that the degree of fatigue went down in the same period. Patients who lived outside the 'envelope' usually experienced deterioration or no improvement (2011).

Several of the newer American self-help books on ME recommend classic pacing, including Bruce Campbell's *Managing Chronic Fatigue Syndrome and Fibromyalgia* (2010) and Erica Verrillo's *Chronic Fatigue Syndrome – A Treatment Guide* (2012). Studies using questionnaires have been done among patients in a number of countries. In these, classic pacing has always shown good results. The method has usually been the one most patients have tried out. Also, the great majority felt that the methods were useful, and very few reported negative effects.

CLASSIC PACING IN NORWAY

In Norway, both ME patient organisations have, from the beginning, recommended classic pacing since they were established in, respectively, 1987 and 1991. The method is also recommended by several professionals, among these the ME/CFS Centre for Adults at Oslo University Hospital, Aker. Irma Pinxterhuis, occupational therapist, has done several studies (2008 and 2011) that have shown that patients at many different functioning levels find classic pacing useful. Live Hareide, psychologist, got the same results (2007) among young people. This is confirmed in a study using a questionnaire among 828 Norwegian people with ME, which was conducted by psychologist Torunn Bjørkum. In this study, 96% of the patients stated that they had good results from pacing. Unfortunately, the questions in the questionnaire did not ask patients to explain what the improvement consisted of. The large study done by the Norwegian ME Association in 2013 confirmed that pacing is useful for the majority of patients.

COGNITIVE BEHAVIOURAL THERAPY AND GRADED EXERCISE THERAPY

In some literature reviews, it is said that Cognitive Behavioural Therapy and Graded Exercise Therapy are the most promising treatments for Chronic Fatigue Syndrome (for example, in the article by Chambers and colleagues (2006) mentioned in the literature list at the back of the book). Both therapies are based on the bio-psychosocial model. This model views illness as an interaction between biological, emotional and social factors. In connection with ME, the model by Jan

Vercoulen (1998) is often referred to. According to this model, a number of factors can trigger Chronic Fatigue Syndrome, but the illness is maintained by behavioural and psychological factors. The theory states that patients have a fear of movement in addition to certain personality traits, including neurotic perfectionism and introversion. This is said to result in the patients doing too little, which weakens muscles and causes discomfort on physical activity. In this model, patients are stuck in a vicious circle where they do less in response to symptoms caused by weakness, because they think they have an ongoing illness.

Based on Vercoulen's model and similar ones, some researchers have recommended Cognitive Behavioural Therapy (CBT) and Graded Exercise Therapy. CBT is a psychological treatment, which aims to teach the patients to recognize negative thought and behavioural patterns, and to change these. When this approach has been used with ME patients, it has usually been based on Vercoulen's or similar models. As a consequence, the patients have been asked to gradually increase activities to work their way out of the fear of movement, which is central to this model. In some cases a different type of CBT has been used. This is described in the paragraph 'Type B CBT', later in this chapter.

Graded Exercise Therapy (GET) involves gradually introducing more physical activity and exercise several times per week, and then continuing to increase it. In ME, the theory behind GET is to increase fitness and muscle mass, which some professionals believe the patients have lost, and to tell the patients that it is not dangerous for them to be physically active.

THE FIRST HYBRID

Hybrids are a mixture of pacing and grading (gradual increase). For this reason they can be described as a mixture of pacing, CBT and GET. I have chosen to call these hybrids because hybrid means a combination of two different elements. The hybrids are aimed at gradually normalising the activity level, whereas classic pacing is about adapting to the limitations imposed on you by the illness. The first hybrid was probably the one that was made by the occupational therapist Dianne Cox, at the hospital at Romford in England in the early 1990s. She later described this in the book *Occupational Therapy and Chronic Fatigue Syndrome* (2000). Here Cox discusses the rationale of CBT and GET, and explains how she combined these to create her own programme. Cox gives some importance to

CHAPTER 22: BACKGROUND AND DISCUSSION

listening to the patients and taking their perceived limitations into account. For this reason her programme also had traits of pacing, even though it was a mixture of CBT and GET.

The first self-help guide to use the word 'pacing' to describe a hybrid programme is called *Chronic Fatigue Syndrome: The Facts*, by Frankie Campling and Michael Sharpe, which was also published in 2000. Campling and Sharpe are among the most well-known advocates of a theory that is very similar to Vercoulen's. Sharpe was also amongst the first to do research on CBT in Chronic Fatigue Syndrome, and is known to heartily recommend this treatment. Even though Campling and Sharpe called their management programme pacing, it mostly resembles Cognitive Behavioural Therapy.

FIGURE 2 – BOOKS ABOUT HYBRID PROGRAMMES

- Frankie Campling and Michael Sharpe, *Chronic Fatigue Syndrome: The Facts*, 2000 and 2008

- Emily Collingridge, *Severe ME/CFS: A Guide to Living*, 2010

- Diane Cox, *Occupational Therapy and Chronic Fatigue Syndrome*, 2000

- Jill Moss, *A Ray of Hope*, 2008

- Sue Pemberton and Catherine Berry, *Fighting Fatigue*, 2009

- Shropshire Enablement Team, *Setting the Pace*, 2009

See the reference list for more information about the books.

MORE ABOUT THE HYBRIDS

There are two types of hybrids, those called pacing or something similar, and those called CBT or GET. In both groups it varies quite a bit how much weight is put on pacing.

Hybrid programmes are characterised by four main traits.

1. They are aimed at any type of chronic fatigue because they assume that the

cause is the same. For this reason they do not separate between groups of patients defined with different diagnostic criteria.

2. They emphasize stability because they believe that ME is maintained by bursts of overactivity, which give symptom flare ups followed by underactivity caused by the belief that activity is harmful.

3. The hybrids recommend stabilizing the activity level by using a detailed activity diary, and a fairly strict daily routine. Diaries and routines are presented as necessities.

4. Great emphasis is placed on increasing the activity level.

The programmes are based on the assumption that increase in activity is necessary to obtain improvement, and that lack of increase will lead to deterioration. Several also assume that the patient cannot feel improvement, and therefore do not increase activity by themselves. According to these programmes, you do not have to wait until symptoms have improved before you increase the activity level. It is enough to wait until the symptoms are stable. Jill Moss (2008) defines stability as the symptoms not being significantly worse. Some do not define how long it takes to stabilise the illness, while others suggest a period of stabilization as short as one to two weeks. It is emphasised that the increase in activity level should be very small and that it is important to not increase too fast. Still, the books commonly suggest that it is possible to increase every week or every second week.

In addition to these four main characteristics, the hybrid programmes also have other traits in common. None of the hybrids that I have detailed information about have given instructions on how to construct a routine based on a detailed activity diary.

In general, the hybrids advise people to continue increasing activities in just about any circumstance and to avoid lowering activity level, even when symptoms occur. Furthermore, hybrids usually give little or no advice on what to do if the first routine you construct turns out not to work out well. An overview of the self-help books which present hybrid programmes can be found in Figure 2.

In Great Britain, the hybrid programmes have become common. A common misunderstanding in that country is that hybrids are pacing, and there is little awareness around the fact that these programmes often only contain some elements of it. In other countries hybrid programmes are a lot less prominent. British patients have told me that there are variations in how British professionals use the hybrids in practice. The use does not only vary from clinic to clinic, but also between professionals working at the same clinic. In reality, this means that patients at some clinics are pressured to increase their activity level faster than they consider viable, while patients at other places have more freedom of choice of speed, even though the aim is always to increase the activity level. This quote by Isla, aged eight, illustrates the problem:

> *"You are meant to understand my illness, but all you do is push, push, push. Nothing I do is ever good enough. I am proud and think you will be pleased with me, as I have been going to school much more than before, but all you do is say I need to stay there longer, and if I feel ill I can't come home early... I don't like coming to see you; it makes me worry what you're going to ask me to do next... I think you should care more about the children who come to see you, and try to understand what they're going through."*

IS VERCOULEN'S MODEL CORRECT?

Vercoulen and colleagues (1998) tested their model on a group of patients, but the study has been criticised because they did not use known diagnostic criteria when including patients in the study. Sharon Song and Leonard Jason (2005) therefore chose to test the model on a range of different fatiguing conditions. Vercoulen's model turned out to be correct for people who had chronic fatigue caused by psychiatric illness. The results indicated that people with chronic fatigue of psychiatric origin had fear of movement combined with personality traits which could perpetuate their symptoms. Vercoulen's model did not fit other types of chronic fatigue, including people with Chronic Fatigue Syndrome defined by the Fukuda criteria. Until recently, the Fukuda criteria were the most commonly used for CFS and ME research studies.

It is not particularly surprising that the model did not fit Chronic Fatigue Syndrome as defined by the Fukuda criteria. Other research studies have shown a range of abnormalities which does not fit with Vercoulen's model. Several of the abnormal results have turned out to be more common after overexertion and exercise. Amongst other things, the researchers Frank Twisk and Michael Maes (2009) mention inflammatory processes, disturbances in the immune system, levels

CHAPTER 22: BACKGROUND AND DISCUSSION

of anti-oxidants that are too low, levels of free radicals that are too high, increased amounts of nitric oxide and peroxynitrite, leaky ion channels in the cell membranes, and defects in the stress response mechanisms.

Most of these results stem from studies using moderately strict criteria. The vast majority of these findings cannot occur as a result of psychological problems, and cannot be exercised away either. On the contrary, they are worsened by exercise. Treatments which prescribe increases in activity level or exercise are likely to have no positive effect for patients with these abnormalities and could even cause damage. This is supported by the fact that Gallagher and colleagues (2005) did not manage to find fear of movement in CFS patients defined by the Oxford criteria and the Fukuda criteria. In this study, some patients fulfilled both the Oxford and the Fukuda criteria, while others only fulfilled the Oxford criteria. None of the patients had additional psychiatric diagnoses. Most patients who had fulfilled the Oxford criteria did not fulfil criteria for ME, and must therefore be assumed to suffer from other illnesses. According to Vercoulen's model, these patients should have a fear of movement. As mentioned above, Gallagher did not find fear of movement in any of the patients, not even those who only fulfilled the Oxford criteria. The results fit in well with Song and Jason's research, which shows that people with other types of physical fatigue than ME did not have fear of movement either. Despite numerous attempts it has not been possible to document personality traits which can perpetuate ME. Vercoulen's model appears to be correct for chronic fatigue in some people; however, this model does not fit other types of chronic fatigue.

DISCUSSION OF PACING

Even though most of the large international research groups support the use of pacing, some professionals have criticised the method. Jill Moss (who is a patient organisation representative and not a health care professional), sums up the criticism in her new book *A Ray of Hope* (2008). According to Moss, pacing has a tendency to be interpreted differently by different people. Moss says that pacing is about continuing with an activity until you get symptoms, and then resting, and that this will lead to a rollercoaster pattern, where the patients do far too much on good days, and then have to rest to recover. Furthermore, the lack of a strict routine will contribute to the patients being overactive on good days. The focus on listening to one's body will mean that the patients expect to feel worse from activity, and this will be a self-fulfilling prophecy. If the patient tries to avoid overexertion by stopping before they get symptoms, they will not increase activity in the long run.

This criticism of pacing has been badly defined and is only partially correct. In the literature, pacing is often described in different ways (e.g. with metaphors). The basic methods are easily recognizable, however, and are the same, or virtually the same, regardless of which country or time period you look at. The variations may be described as a strength because they make pacing relevant to different subgroups of patients. The patients will have different circumstances, and it will be possible to adapt the management programme to each individual.

Moss claims that pacing causes a rollercoaster pattern. The allegation seems strange as books about classic pacing stress that this is the very pattern which pacing is meant to prevent. This includes Moss' own book from 1995. Judging from the description in this and other books, doing too much on good days and then resting to recover equals lack of pacing. Using a strict routine does not necessarily prevent overexertion on good days. Several patients have told me that the lack of spontaneity in such routines can make it very tempting to plunge yourself head first into something you know you are not well enough for, while a somewhat more flexible programme can counteract this urge. The allegation that the patients do not increase activity if they stop before they get symptoms, suggest that patients cannot feel that they are getting better. Research on classic pacing, such as the study by Molly Brown and Leonard Jason, which was mentioned earlier in this chapter, shows that the patients can feel that they are getting better, and increase activity themselves when they are well enough for it. This however, is true for people with quite strictly defined ME.

For people with chronic fatigue as a result of psychological disease, the situation is different. The allegation that pacing can lead to a gradual decline in activity level makes sense according to Vercoulen's model. Advocates of this model have pointed out that people with a fear of movement have a tendency to over-interpret normal physical signals from the body, thinking they are signs of illness. For these patients, learning to stop before they get symptoms may possibly lead to a slow downhill spiral in activity level. Pacing is therefore not necessarily a good approach for people with chronic fatigue as a result of psychiatric illness.

DISCUSSION OF CBT AND GET

In some of the CBT and GET studies, the patients have been selected using the Oxford criteria. In these studies some patients usually get better whereas others get worse, and a third group has no effect. Dropout rates have usually been high, and the researchers have rarely accounted for the reasons why the patients ended the treatment. In addition, the studies have usually been of short duration, and the patients have often not been followed up afterwards. Most of the studies have not used objective measurements of activity level before, during and after treatment.

In a study by Black and colleagues in 2005, where such measures were used, the researchers found that the patients, only a few days into the study, had to reduce other activities to keep up the exercise. The unfit, healthy controls could increase activity level with no problem. The researchers therefore concluded that exercise does not improve the illness.

All of these aspects have contributed to much criticism of the CBT and GET studies. The method used in CBT and GET is aimed at treating fear of movement and deconditioning. As mentioned in the paragraph 'Is Vercoulen's Model Correct?' fear of movement has not been found in patients with chronic fatigue of physical origin, whereas this was found in chronic fatigue of psychological origin. The variations in the results of the effect from the CBT and GET trials is probably the result of the fact that the Oxford criteria are very unspecific and define a very varied group of patients. All one can conclude from these studies is that CBT and GET are suitable for some people with chronic fatigue as a general phenomenon, but by no means for everyone.

It is a pity that no one has carried out controlled trials of these treatments on sub-groups of chronic fatigue, particularly people with chronic fatigue as a result of psychological illness. Without such studies it is impossible to say who, if any, these treatments are suitable for. It does however seem reasonable to assume that the treatments are suitable for some people who have the problems these treatments were designed to treat, that is people with chronic fatigue of psychiatric origin.

For people with strictly defined neurological ME, there is significant evidence that these treatments are unsuitable (an overview of this can be found in an article by Twisk and Maes). For instance, there have been numerous findings which explain the patients' low functional level and considerable exercise intolerance. This has made a number of researchers question the use of forms of treatment which involve gradual increase of activities. Based on results from biomedical research, research on CBT and GET, and patient surveys, Frank Twisk and Michael Maes (2009) conclude that *"...not only is the evidence based claims for CBT/GET unjust, there is compelling evidence that CBT/GET is potentially harmful for many ME/CFS patients."* (p. 295). They continue *"...therefore it is medically unethical to subject ME/CFS patients to CBT/GET programmes or variants like GET with limits (Nijs et al 2008) without assessing biological abnormalities, monitoring functional impairment objectively and measuring the effect of exercise e.g. on the physical and neurocognitive performance (e.g. by using exercise tests/re-tests, measurements, blood analysis and neurocognitive tests)."*

In summary, it appears that CBT and GET can be of value in fatigue of psychiatric origin, but that the treatments can be poorly suited and potentially damaging to the health of patients with strictly defined ME.

TYPE B CBT

Please note that some of the CBT programmes used in ME are not based on Vercoulen's model, nor train the patients in graded activity/exercise. Such programmes are based on the idea of ME as a physical illness which gives actual limitations, and the aim is to teach the patients to manage the illness as well as possible. These CBT programmes are reminiscent of those used in other chronic physical illnesses. In some reviews of research articles on Chronic Fatigue Syndrome, these programmes have been called 'Type B CBT'. The programmes based on Vercoulen's model, and which contain graded activity, are called 'Type A'. The vast majority of the CBT studies which have been published have been Type A.

One example of a Type B programme is an internet-based programme the American psychologist Bruce Campbell started at the end of the 1990s. In Campbell's programme, classic pacing is taught. The patients were satisfied with the programme, and it still exists. The programme is now called a self-help course. Campbell probably changed the name to avoid confusion with Type A CBT. The vast majority of CBT programmes which have been published in peer-review journals have been Type A. When I talk about CBT in this chapter, I refer to Type

A, unless otherwise stated.

In Norway, the psychologists Torkil Berge and Lars Dehli have used a Type B CBT programme, which they have described in the peer-review article *Kognitiv terapi ved kronisk utmattelsessyndrom og ME* (Cognitive Therapy in Chronic Fatigue Syndrome and ME) and in the self-help book *Energityvene: Utmattelse i sykdom og hverdag* (The Energy Thieves: Fatigue in Illness and in Everyday Life), which they wrote in collaboration with the psychologist Elin Fjerstad. They write explicitly that their programme is based on the CBT programmes used in other physical illnesses. The activity management part of their programme is, however, a hybrid which they call GET. The way the authors describe the programme they use is as a form of structured pacing. This is a good example of the confusion of terminology described earlier.

DISCUSSION OF HYBRID PROGRAMMES

What about the hybrids? Do they suit everyone since they appear to be a compromise? There has been little research on hybrid programmes, at least under the names 'pacing', 'activity management', 'fatigue management' and 'energy management'. These are amongst the names of hybrid programmes used at British clinics. Research on hybrids called CBT and GET are difficult to separate from pure CBT and GET studies. In a study published by Peter White and colleagues (2011), a hybrid called 'adaptive pacing therapy' was used. In this study, however, the patients were defined using the Oxford criteria, which means that this study cannot be compared to the range of studies where other criteria were used. Research has not provided any clear answers as to which hybrid methods may be helpful for which subgroup of chronic fatigue. Because the techniques have not been systematically tested on different subgroups, it is not possible to say what effect the treatments had on any specific group of patients. What we are left with are results from patient surveys, plus patient experiences, normally collected by the patient organisations.

Amongst the patient surveys I have had access to or seen referred to, only three have asked specifically about hybrids. One was Action for ME's survey amongst Scottish members from 2007, where they asked about people's experiences with graded activity. This is one of the names used on some hybrid programmes. Graded activity is not the same as graded exercise, but a similar programme where the focus is on increasing the total activity level. According to Twisk and Maes, Action for ME found that 54% had become worse from graded activity. 14% of the patients experienced no effect from the programme, whereas 32% found it helpful. In 2010, Action for ME carried out another membership survey, this time about the effect of different types of physical therapy. Sixty six patients replied that they had tried graded activity. Of these, 39.4% reported some degree of improvement, while 31% experienced no effect and 26.3% got worse. The difference between the patients who got better and those who got worse were statistically significant, but it is worrying that most of the patients who reported worsening of their illness became much worse (10.5%) or very much worse (13.2%). Only one person (2.6%) reported that their health became only a bit worse.

In the Norwegian ME Association's large patient survey, which was completed in 2013, patients were asked about a wide range of treatments, including a treatment by the CFS/ME team at the children's clinic at the University Hospital of Oslo. This clinic uses a hybrid programme based on strict activity plans. Of the 30 patients who answered that they had received treatment at the clinic, 27% said that they had varying degrees of deterioration, while 10% said that they had improved. No one experienced great improvement. The remaining 63% had no changes in health. The low number of patients who have tried this treatment means that one cannot draw definite conclusions. Besides, the results cannot be generalized to all hybrid programmes. Still, there is nothing about the results of the three hybrid programme surveys which indicates that this treatment is suitable for everyone.

This impression is confirmed by stories from people with moderately to strictly defined ME. In the cases where the patients benefited from the programme, one is often left with the impression that it was the pacing part of the programme which made the patient better, not the gradual increase in activity, which is actually the aim of the programme. In *InterAction*, Action for ME's membership newsletter, July 2002, Abigail Owen tells of her stay at a special unit at the hospital in Romford, which uses Diane Cox's programme. Owen writes that the first thing the staff at the ward did was to give her an activity plan where she was supposed to do half of what she normally did at home. She also explains that she had never before had the opportunity to ask somebody for help to get to the toilet, and that she chose to make full use of the services of the nursing staff. On the fourth day at the hospital, Owen woke up without a headache and a sore throat for the first time in seven years.

She writes that the programme at the hospital gave her body the opportunity to heal. When she wrote the article two and a half years after her hospital stay, her functional ability had considerably improved, but she still had a significant degree of functional impairment.

In Owen's case, it seems obvious that it was the increased amount of rest at the start of the programme which kick-started the gradual improvement and enabled her to keep up when the amount of activity was increased. Furthermore, it is not surprising that she managed to keep up with the increases at first since she started at a level which was only half of what she normally did at home. I have read of a number of similar cases where it seems that an increase in rest made the difference. Some of these stories were about programmes which were given names other than pacing.

Owen also writes: *"Not everyone on the ward with me was lucky; some did not benefit and I witnessed others who actually deteriorated in a hospital environment."* As Owen points out, some people may have become worse because they were in a hospital with noise and other stimulation, but there are also several other possible reasons why people with strictly defined neurological ME, who try hybrid programmes, may not get better. It could be that some need medical treatment they do not get, such as treatment of active infections. However, lack of improvement may also be due to the programme itself. As mentioned in the paragraph about hybrid programmes, some books recommend that one does not lower the activity level to any particular degree. This means that not everyone will get so much rest that it kick-starts natural improvement, like in Owen's case.

In addition, the short stabilization period and the strong focus on increases in activity may lead to the patients being asked to increase the activity level too early and too quickly. This can in turn result in overexertion and relapse. Another weakness of the hybrid programmes is that they rarely assess the risk of deterioration in the individual patient before the patients are asked to increase their activity level. This means that factors like the degree of illness stability and severity may not be taken into account. The same is true for other factors which may negatively impact the patient's health. This too can result in the danger of overactivity. The structure of hybrid programmes is strongly reminiscent of the structure of CBT and GET programmes. This means that there is a risk that a programme which is meant to have noticeable focus on pacing may slide into a programme of enforced activity with a steadily increasing effort load.

The study by Brown, Khorana and Jason, which was mentioned in the paragraph 'Classic Pacing in Different Countries' suggests that it is pacing that makes it possible to increase the activity level. In that case, it can be detrimental to use management programmes which carry with them a risk of the patients overexerting themselves, particularly because it is so well documented that overactivity can be harmful in ME.

Is there a real danger of overactivity in hybrid programmes when you have strictly defined neurological ME? In hybrid programmes increases in activity are compulsory. Sometimes exercise is also compulsory. It does vary how early and quickly the patients are asked to increase their activity level, but all the same, the main focus is on increasing the activity level. To improve the health of the patients, it is necessary to have programmes which are unambiguous and counteract overexertion. It will be counterproductive to use programmes in which activity increase and sometimes exercise are compulsory, which is true for both the hybrid programmes CBT and GET. I have to conclude that hybrid programmes do indeed involve a real danger of overactivity.

The objections listed above are true for people with strictly defined neurological ME who do not have additional psychiatric diagnoses. The situation is different for people with chronic fatigue as a result of psychiatric illness. Here one must ask whether hybrid programmes put too much emphasis on pacing, or whether they put too little emphasis on dealing with the psychiatric problems which are the cause of the patient's illness.

It is also possible that hybrid programmes will have a good effect on a third group of patients: those with fatigue of a physical origin, who also have significant psychological factors. It is possible that some of these develop fear of movement, and that hybrid programmes could have some positive effect on this group of patients, because some of the hybrids, at least in theory, take account of emotional as well as physical factors.

Even though hybrid programmes appear to be a compromise between pacing, CBT and GET, there is much to indicate that they will only be optimal for a small minority of patients with chronic fatigue as a general phenomenon. For others, perhaps the majority of patients with chronic fatigue, hybrids may be poorly adapted, and could at worst be detrimental.

CONCLUSION

This book is aimed at people with strictly defined neurological ME, not chronic fatigue in general. Based on the analysis in this chapter, I have chosen to present classic pacing. Since it is now well documented that exercise with overactivity can worsen the disease process in strictly defined neurological ME, it is my opinion that it is completely necessary that management programmes used in the illness aim to prevent overactivity. Classic pacing is therefore well suited to this. In classic pacing, the focus is on staying within one's energy limits at all stages and levels of illness, including when one is in a phase of improvement and can increase activity. Furthermore, it is my opinion that it is a huge advantage that classic pacing is not linked to certain strategies, but can be adapted to each individual's life situation. This increases the probability that the patients are capable of using the method. Even though little research has been carried out on classic pacing, the research that has been published shows that we have every reason to continue investigating the method. Patient surveys are unanimous: Pacing and rest are the interventions from which the most patients report benefit. This corresponds with the experience of many healthcare professionals and is supported by research on pacing and by biochemical research on ME in general. In her article, *Erfaringer med pleie i institusjon ved alvorlig ME* (Experiences with Institutional Care in severe Myalgic Encephalopathy) in the peer reviewed journal *Norsk Tidsskrift for Sykepleieforskning* (Norwegian Journal of Nursing Research), the experienced ME doctor and pathologist Sidsel Kreyberg writes: *"Experience must, for now, be accepted as key to understanding and managing this largely unexplained disorder."* For this reason it is the patients' experiences that have formed the basis for this book.

CHAPTER 23:

TIPS FOR ENERGY CONSERVATION

INTRODUCTION

Some of the tips in this chapter are easy to carry out while others require more work. Some of them you will like straight away, while others may not suit you at all. In some countries it is possible to borrow aids like shower stools and wheelchairs from the National Health Service or voluntary organisations. If this is the case, there is no need to spend money on buying everything yourself. Make a list of your ten favourite tips and introduce them in a tempo which feels suitable. When you have started using all the tips, you can read the chapter again and perhaps choose another ten suggestions. It is also possible to create energy conservation tips of your own. You can think through what you normally do, and how this can be done in a less strenuous way. Turn it into a game.

KITCHEN

- A standing support chair or perching stool saves a lot of energy because you can sit in situations where people normally stand. It may be possible to borrow this from the National Health Service.

- Kitchen supplies which are frequently used should be placed within easy reach.

- When possible, choose lightweight kitchen equipment. There are many types of kitchen equipment with thick handles which are easier to hold such as cheese cutters.

- Use a food processor if you need to cut up a large amount of vegetables. When the amounts are small, it is easier to use a knife.

- Make extra portions when you cook. Extra portions can be frozen in numbered plastic containers. Many dishes are well suited for freezing, especially those with

CHAPTER 23: TIPS FOR ENERGY CONSERVATION

a lot of sauce. It is a good idea to make extra sauce, as some of the moisture will evaporate during thawing. You can freeze different accompaniments, such as potatoes and vegetables in the same containers, so that you get several home-made convenience foods. Accessories can also be made separately and frozen, or put in the fridge. Single people can cook four portions of food, twice a week, and re-heat home-made convenience foods the other days. After a few weeks, you will have a variety of frozen dishes to choose from.

- Quick dishes require less energy to make. You can get special cook books for quick dishes.

- It may be possible for you to have others prepare large amounts of food for you to eat. Shop-bought convenience foods also save energy, but this may not be suitable for people with food intolerances.

- In some areas there is a community 'meals on wheels' service, but this food may require extra spices to become tasty.

SHOPPING

- Create a standard shopping list of things you need every week.

- Order food online, or at a local supermarket once a month, so that you need to buy less every week. Even in the middle of big cities you may find local grocery stores that deliver to people in their area.

- Use a wheeled shopper or a backpack instead of plastic bags when you go shopping.

- A 'featherweight' camping stool or a seat stick are useful if you have difficulty waiting in line. Seat sticks, or shooting sticks, often come with a small bag so that you do not need to hold it in your hand all the time.

- Try shopping at a time when there are fewer people in the shop.

CLEANING

- Get a cleaner or carer if possible.

- It is easier to deal with cleaning and tidying if you do a little frequently, rather than waiting until there is a lot of dirt or mess. This involves putting things away as soon as you have used them. Similarly, you can wipe small spots of the bathroom mirror instead of waiting until you have to wash the whole thing.

- If you are doing cleaning for yourself, split the cleaning into small bits. For instance, clean the sink at one time, and the toilet later that day, or the next day.

- A lot of cleaning can be done sitting on a chair with wheels, including vacuum cleaning.

- Noisy jobs (such as vacuuming) can be less strenuous if you wear ear plugs.

- Dry mopping is less strenuous in every way compared to vacuuming.

- Modern microfibre products are easy to use because you do not need soap with them, so you avoid the strong smell of cleaning agents.

- When soap is necessary, you can use unperfumed varieties.

- Scrubbing sponges save energy because you do not have to rub as hard as you do with a wash cloth. You can also try the stain removing sponges 'Swiffer Magic' or 'Scotch Bright'.

- Furniture on wheels makes cleaning easier. You can buy wheels that can be screwed on to the furniture, such as the legs of the sofa table. The best is to get wheels with brakes, because this enables you to choose when the piece of furniture should stand still, and when it should be movable.

MEALS

- You may find cutlery with thick handles easier to hold – these can be bought in shops that sell small aids for disabled people.

- Plastic cutlery and plates makes less noise and are suitable for people with severe sensitivity to noise.

- Plastic glasses and cups weigh considerably less than products made from glass or porcelain.

- When you use a straw you do not need to lift the cup to your mouth.

- Hot drinks can be kept in a pump action thermos flask. This type of flask can also be used to keep cold drinks cold.

- A flexible arm with a cup holder can make it possible for you to drink by yourself even if you cannot hold the cup. These can be bought from shops that sell aids for disabled people.

- The drinking bottle 'The Hydrant' has a sucking tube which makes it possible to drink lying down without having to lift anything except the lightweight tube. The tube can also be fastened to a pillow with a clip, which enables you to drink just by turning your head. Available from www.hydrateforhealth.co.uk.

- You can also use a 'Camelback' drinking bag, which is available at sports shops, but these are harder to clean. The water in the bag should be changed often. When using the Camelback bag or The Hydrant it is important to get a cleaning kit with a long brush so that you can clean the tube properly.

- Sandwiches can be put in lunch boxes next to the bed.

- Soft food is easier to chew.

- It is easier to eat from a bowl with a spoon than from a flat plate using a knife and fork. This is particularly true if you raise the table a little so that the distance from the table to the mouth becomes smaller. Bed tables which stand on the floor are height adjustable.

- Others can assist you by cutting up your food. You can also choose dishes that do not need to be cut.

- Most food can be puréed down and thinned so that they can be drunk through thick straws. When you thin puréed food with water you get a higher volume with the same calories, so make sure you are still getting enough calories. Alternatively, you can thin the food with something which contains calories, for instance sauce, stock, juice, milk or custard.

- Puréed food and soup can be poured into thermal mugs. The lightest thermal mugs only keep the contents hot for an hour, but some of the moderate weight ones can keep the food hot for six hours.

- If you become so weak that you can only eat liquid food, it is vitally important not to live off SlimFast or similar weight loss products. In the long run this will lead to severe malnutrition. Instead, it is better to drink home-made thinned purée or nutritional drinks from the pharmacy, which are meant to be used as sole source of nutrition.

- In the rare cases that people get so weak that they do not get enough food, it can help to have a tube inserted in the nose to the stomach so that you can have liquid feed pumped directly into your stomach. This saves a lot of energy and prevents weight loss.

CHAPTER 23: TIPS FOR ENERGY CONSERVATION

- There are many different types of tube feed, including types suitable for different types of food intolerance.

- If you have an unusually high number of food intolerances, it may, however, be difficult to find a feed you can tolerate. Then it may be possible to have a tube inserted surgically into the duodenum, a so-called PEG tube. This tube is so wide you can pour in puréed food with porridge-like consistency. It is fully possible to pour in home-made food, which enables you to adapt the diet to your own needs.

BATHROOM

- A lightweight shower stool can be lifted out of the shower and placed in front of the sink so that you can wash sitting down.

- A bath board is a seat that goes across the bathtub.

- If you mount a pull out shaving mirror at sitting height, you can brush your teeth, put on make-up and shave sitting down.

- An electric toothbrush saves energy, but some people have problems with the vibrations.

- After bathing or showering you can put on a terry bathrobe and only dry your face and feet. Then you might as well rest in the bathrobe for a while before you get dressed.

- An inflatable hair washbasin makes it possible to have your hair washed in bed. Available from shops that sell care products.

- Use shampoo and conditioner in one, or just use shampoo.

- Hair can be blow-dried lying flat in bed with the hair hanging over the edge of the bed. The person who is drying your hair for you can then sit on a chair next to you.

- Use ear plugs when blow-drying your hair.

- Let your hair air dry if possible.

- Short hair is easier to wash and dry than long hair, but has to be cut more often.

- Hands-free holders for hairdryers are available. To see the different types, do an Internet search for 'Hands-free hairdryer holder'.

- Choose an easily kept hairstyle that demands as little work as possible.

295

- A commode next to the bed is a possibility if you have difficulty walking to the toilet.

- You can also use a bed pan or urinal bottle. Urinal bottles are available in both male and female versions.

- See also the next section on freedom of movement if you have difficulty getting to and from the toilet.

FREEDOM OF MOVEMENT

- A mobility scooter or an electric wheelchair gives you a freedom of movement you can otherwise only dream about.

- Indoors, an electrically powered office chair may be better than an ordinary wheelchair, because it takes up less space and requires a smaller turning circle.

- You can scoot yourself around sitting on an office chair or on the seat of a rollator. It is easier to scoot yourself backwards and to push yourself forwards.

- Some benefit from walking aids like crutches, sticks, Nordic walking sticks or a rollator. Nordic walking sticks are similar to ski sticks, and are normally used to increase the exercise benefit of walking. They can be bought from sport shops. It is usually symptoms like pain, weakness and unsteadiness which necessitate the use of various walking aids. These symptoms may be a sign of overexertion. For this reason it is important not to use walking aids to push yourself to walk as far as possible. Instead, they should be used to walk short distances in a way that is as comfortable as possible. Use a wheelchair or car for longer distances.

- Using walking aids and manual wheelchairs puts a strain on the arms. Be careful not to overexert your arms.

- Car travel is less exhausting if you lie in the back seat or sit in the passenger seat with the back reclined.

- Ear plugs, ear defenders and eye masks reduce motion sickness.

- If you are dizzy and walk unsteadily, using ear plugs may help.

READING, WRITING AND COMMUNICATION

- Large print is easier to read. Adjust your computer so that it automatically writes with large letters, and borrow large-print books from the library.

- A variety of newspapers and magazines are available in audio format. For some, audio books are easier to concentrate on. Audio books are expensive but can be borrowed at the library. Most countries have audio libraries for people with vision and reading problems. You usually need a note from your doctor to access this library.

- School books are available in audio format. Ask a special education teacher or an educational psychologist how to obtain these in your country.

- Many different book holders are available, which enable you to read without having to hold the book. These can be bought from shops that sell aids for disabled people or possibly be borrowed from the National Health Service or voluntary organisations.

- Many find it easier to type on a computer than to write by hand, particularly if you have a laptop computer which can be used in bed or on the sofa.

- Use thick pens with balls that roll easily. Ink pens, gel pens and mechanical pencils create less friction than ballpoint pens and regular pencils.

- It is also possible to record what you want to write on a Dictaphone and then get others to type it out afterwards.

- Different types of computer mice and keyboards plus holders for laptop computers can make it easier to use a computer.

- There are programs which enlarge the text on the screen or read the text back to you.

- Dictation programmes are discussed in the paragraph about writing problems in Chapter 17, 'Learning, School and Studies'.

- Internet forums of the message board type require less energy than the ones where you chat in real time.

- If you have difficulty typing texts, it may help to get a phone with a touch screen, which requires less energy than buttons.

- It is possible to record sound MMSs and send to other people, but not all phones can receive each other's messages.

- Several mobiles now have inbuilt programmes which write down what you say. The precision is not always so good, but it is expected that it will improve with time. There are several different dictation apps available, some of which are free, and several of these are better than the inbuilt systems.

- Many mobiles have functions which read the text from the screen out loud. On other mobiles you can download apps which do this.

- Some mobiles have a function which enlarges the text on the screen.

- Most modern smartphones can understand voice commands, such as "Phone John".

- Video calls, either on the mobile or on Skype, may be easier to concentrate on than normal phone calls.

- If you have speech problems, you can spell what you want to say by pointing on an alphabet board or on a board containing the words you use the most, for instance 'food', 'drink', 'toilet', etc. A board like this can also be made with pictures instead of words.

- Both simple and advanced speech machines are available for disabled people. In some countries it may be possible to borrow these from the National Health Service.

- Voice amplifiers are available if you can only whisper.

- In *Surviving Severe ME*, Claire Wade suggests the following system of communication: Moving the thumb means 'yes', the little finger 'no', the second finger 'food', the middle finger 'drink', and the ring finger 'toilet'. You can speak in the dark if your assistant feels for your hand.

- Blowing or blinking can be used as a signal for 'yes'. This enables you to reply to simple yes-no questions such as 'toilet?'.

- If you communicate via written notes, you can have the most common messages written out on small cards so that you do not have to write them again every time.

SENSORY SENSITIVITY

- When there is noise from building work or road work, it is best to go away if possible.

- Use double hearing protection (both ear plugs and ear defenders) if you have to stay at home.

- There are many different types of both ear plugs and ear defenders.

- Cylindrical foam ear plugs which are rough on the outside tend to make your ears less sore if you have to wear them for a long time. These, however, do not give the strongest hearing protection.

- Light can be softened with sunglasses, baseball cap, blinds and blackout curtains, which can also be sewn into normal curtains.

- Lamplights can be softened with low powered lightbulbs and good shades. Fairy lights may be suitable to get a low light.

- To minimize vibrations from wheelchairs and cars it is important to have good cushioning, good springs and an even surface.

- It is possible to get vibration minimizing rubber cups, which can be put under the feet of washing machines and dryers.

- Furniture pads made from felt and rubber can be placed under the feet of furniture to reduce vibration and noise. They can also be put on the inside of cupboard doors etc.

- If you are hypersensitive to touch, you can use soft clothes, pressure relief mattress, lightweight duvet, and a special metal contraption, called a bed cradle, which lifts the duvet up from the body.

- Sensitivity to taste can only be alleviated by choosing food and drink which are less problematic (e.g. bland foods).

- If you have difficulty with food smells, it helps to close all internal doors and open the windows.

- Sensitivity to other smells can be helped by using unperfumed products for skin care, cleaning and laundry.

- So called acoustic boards (also called acoustic panels and acoustic ceiling tiles) are used for muffling noise in music studios and kindergartens. You get the effect by hanging them from the ceiling with a few centimetres of air between the ceiling and boards, or by hanging them on the wall with so called distance brackets. Avoid the type which is hung on the wall using spray mount, particularly if you are sensitive to chemicals. For more information, see websites like www.acousticalsolutions.com.

- Solid wooden doors muffle sound better than light doors. You can also get special sound isolating doors, but some of these release chemicals.

APPENDIX

RELAXATION RESOURCES

BOOKS

There is currently a wide range of books available on the subject of relaxation. One that is particularly useful is the prize-winning book *Mindfulness for Health: A Practical Guide to Relieving Pain, Reducing Stress and Restoring Wellbeing* by Vidyamala Burch and Danny Penman. This book contains a lot of information on how to relax in spite of pain, and it comes with a CD with eight relaxation sessions. The CD has no background music, which makes it less tiring to listen to.

COURSES

Relaxation courses are often available at health clubs, yoga centres, pain clinics, and patient support groups. There may be a local information service which can help you find out what is available in your community. Breathworks is a non-profit company which offers relaxation courses in a number of countries around the world, including the UK, Ireland, Germany, the Netherlands, Belgium, Portugal, Italy, Spain and Australia, and soon in Sweden and Turkey. There is also an online course that is available anywhere. Have a look at www.breathworks-mindfulness.org.uk for more information. Many healthcare professionals know how to teach relaxation. This can be useful, as learning relaxation with a teacher is sometimes more effective than trying to learn it on your own, particularly if you are very tense.

CDs

There are many different relaxation CDs available. They can be bought from shops that sell CDs, such as www.amazon.com and www.cdbaby.com. Other sources include yoga centres and patient support groups. Many CDs have background music. This can be useful if you are very stressed, but it can also be too tiring – especially if you are severely affected. Some webpages allow you to hear a short clip of the CD prior to ordering. Please note that some meditation CDs are music only. Guided relaxation generally provides a deeper effect, particularly if you are a

RELAXATION RESOURCES

beginner. If you like CDs with the music only, the webpage www.newworldmusic.com has an amazing range. They also sell some guided CDs with background music.

DOWNLOADS AND PODCASTS

There is a wealth of relaxation tracks available to download online, both from various individual webpages and from sites like www.iTunes.com. Some tracks and series cost money, but there are so many free series available that you are unlikely to ever need to pay anything. Useful search words include 'free relaxation podcasts', 'free meditation podcasts' and 'free mindfulness podcasts'. Adding the word 'guided', such as 'free guided relaxation podcasts', can narrow the search down so that you do not get as many music-only tracks. Below is a list of free series available on iTunes. The list is not exhaustive. Many more are available.

NAME	AVAILABLE FROM
'30 day Relaxation Plan Hypnosis Course' '7 day Cure Insomnia Hypnosis Course'	iTunes.com, JasonNewland.com
'Relaxation by Inner Health Studio'	iTunes.com, InnerHealthStudio.com
'Meditation Oasis'	iTunes.com, MeditationOasis.com
'The Meditation Podcast'	iTunes.com, TheMeditationPodcast.com
'Meditation for Health Podcast'	iTunes.com, MeditationforHealthPodcast.com

SMARTPHONE APPS

Smartphone relaxation apps fall into two groups: those that are free and those that cost a little money to download. Some of the free ones are entirely free, whereas others have a number of free tracks and some you have to pay for. Occasionally, there are very few free tracks, and you have to pay a subscription to access the app. This may cost more than the price of an app that costs money to download. However, the range of free tracks and entirely free apps is so great that you may never need to pay. Please note that some apps stream their content from the Internet to avoid taking up too much memory space on your phone. If this is the case, it can be a good idea to download some of the sessions onto your phone so

303

that you can access them when you do not have Internet access or when Internet access is not free. If your app does not allow for this, you can download some of the free tracks mentioned under 'Downloads and Podcasts'.

To download an app, follow the simple steps below.

1. Go to the app store suitable for your smartphone.

2. Search for relaxation apps. Useful search words include 'relaxation', 'mindfulness' and 'meditation'.

3. Choose the app you want to install. I suggest you start with a free one. If you do not like it, you can always uninstall it and try another one.

FREE RELAXATION APPS:

NAME	BACKGROUND MUSIC	PHONE TYPE	COMMENT
Qigong Meditation Relaxation	Optional	Android	Teaches techniques to cope with discomfort
Calm	Optional	Android /Apple	Sessions vary in length from 3 to 30 minutes
Stop Breathe & Think: Meditate	No	Android /Apple	Motivates you to practise every day
Guided Meditations Free App	Yes	Android	Large number of sessions
iSleep Easy Meditations Free	Optional	Android /Apple	Good sleep help
Relax Lite: Stress Relief	Optional	Android /Apple	Good deep breathing exercises
Insight Timer	Optional	Android/Apple	An amazing number of available tracks

There are very few relaxation apps for Blackberry phones. To compensate, you can download the app 'Sync for iTunes' and use this to transfer free podcasts from iTunes to your phone.

PATHFINDER TO MOVEMENT RESOURCES FOR PEOPLE WITH ME

Not all of the movement systems mentioned below are specially adapted for people with ME. It has not been possible to check the quality of all the listed resources. They are not mentioned as a recommendation, but only to make it easy for the reader to acquire more information on their own. It is essential to find out about the different types of movement before you try one of them, not just to assess which one will work best but also to find out if you are at all well enough to try any of them.

GENTLE YOGA

Several yoga teachers have made programmes specifically for people with ME. Although they are all gentle, the intensity does vary considerably, so do check that the programme suits your ability level.

CDs

Angela Stevens: *Energise and Relax with Yoga*

This super gentle programme is designed to be used lying flat in bed. It is so gentle that it would be a relaxation exercise for people who are healthy. This programme is suitable for people who are quite ill but whose health is improving.

Angela Stevens: *Yoga the Gentle Way*

Though still very gentle, this programme is one step more exerting than *Energise and Relax with Yoga*. It is done lying on the floor. The CD has no background music.

Available from www.angela-stevens.co.uk

Diana Lampen: *For Those with ME*

These lying and sitting exercises require more energy than *Yoga the Gentle Way* by Angela Stevens. It is a long programme, so it is best done in smaller bits. With background music.

Diana Lampen: *ME follow-on tape/cd*

This is aimed at people who have used *For Those with ME* and whose health has improved enough for them to want something more demanding. Diana Lampen also has a range of other CDs, including several relaxation CDs, one of which is for children.

Available from www.hopeproject.co.uk

BOOK

Fiona Agombar: *Beat Fatigue with Yoga*

This book is written by a yoga teacher who has ME herself. Available from www.fionaagombar.co.uk and Internet bookshops.

DVD

Fiona Agombar: *Beat Fatigue with Yoga*

This yoga-DVD contains three sessions of varying degrees of intensity. The gentlest of which is suitable as a follow-on to Angela Stevens' CD, *Yoga the Gentle Way*.

YOUTUBE VIDEOS

There are many yoga videos on YouTube, some of which are suitable for people with ME. The two below were made specifically for the ME/CFS community, which is a part of the CFS Knowledge Centre. The links are very long, but you can find the videos very easily by searching for 'CFS Knowledge Centre'.

Wheelchair Yoga for Those with Severe Physical Limitations – this is a sitting session, mostly consisting of arm movements:

www.youtube.com/watch?v=01kA5qF7mtY&feature=youtu.be

Yoga for Those with Physical Limitations – this session is done on the floor, and many of the exercises can be done lying down:

www.youtube.com/watch?v=mBg-WOvmhJM&feature=youtu.be

YOGA GROUPS

Many local ME groups organise yoga sessions adapted to suit their needs. Please contact your local ME group to find out if this applies to your area. Yoga centres, Buddhist centres and the like may well have sessions adapted to people who need a gentle approach.

QIGONG

DVD

Practising Qigong with Merete Sparre

This video features Merete Sparre, a Norwegian physiotherapist and Qigong instructor who has ME herself. She has used the five exercises in this DVD with hundreds of people with ME. The DVD has no verbal instructions, and is therefore suitable for speakers of any language. The exercises are done standing up, but some of them can be done sitting on a stool. Suitable for people with mild to moderate ME.

Available from www.tropos.no

YOUTUBE VIDEOS

There are a large number of Qigong videos on YouTube, but most of these appear to be standing exercises, often done with the arms outstretched or held over the head for long periods of time. The two videos below are more suited to people with ME. One of them consists of finger exercises and the other one is a programme done lying down. The first exercise consists of holding the arms in the air for 4 minutes. Skip this or reduce it to a few, comfortable seconds. The other exercises are much gentler.

Finger Qigong – Exercises for Chi Circulation in the Fingers:

www.youtube.com/watch?v=7P9EiooL3Ck&list=PL7C6F8ILavYfezkgKOHhl_Cs yzZRJ61WM&index=10

Lying Down Qigong and T'ai Chi Ch'uan (Tai Chi):

www.youtube.com/watch?v=fpA4aWjI_HU&index=3&list=PL_7IJVpWEORqU NT05UABXb4eH-o1KXQUT

QIGONG GROUPS

Group sessions can be found at local tai-chi centres, but be aware that qigong teachers like Merete Sparre use a much gentler version of qigong than what is commonly used at centres. You may not be able to cope with a normal session. Gentle sessions may be available.

BASIC BODY AWARENESS THERAPY

This physiotherapy technique is commonly used in some countries, but is virtually unknown in others. The physiotherapy website, www.gomobilus.com lists the countries in which the method is used. If you live in one of these countries, you can contact your local physiotherapy union to find out how to find a physiotherapist who is familiar with the method. The method may not be in common use, even if it does exist in your country. I have not been able to find any patient-oriented resources in English.

THE ALEXANDER TECHNIQUE

The Alexander Technique combines relaxation and good posture to enable people to let go of their tension and move around with the least amount of energy expenditure.

BOOK

Angela Bradshaw – *Be in Balance.* Balloon View Limited, 2014. ISBN: 978-1-907798-34-4

This fully illustrated, easy-to-read book gives an introduction to the Alexander Technique. Available from Internet bookshops.

VIDEOS

The following three videos are all introductions to the Alexander Technique. The first is the shortest, and is therefore a good place to start:

Angela Bradshaw: *"Show Me How" – The Alexander Technique*:

www.youtube.com/watch?v=prN9kbDtedc

Marjorie Barstow: *Introduction to the Alexander Technique*:

www.youtube.com/watch?v=NdrP_XGEuWI

Ofir Mizrahi: *An Introduction to the Alexander Technique*:

www.youtube.com/watch?v=2hUoEbiskuo

LESSONS

These websites give you general information and allow you to search for a teacher in your area.
www.alexandertechnique.com
www.alexandertechnique.co.uk

REFERENCES

All quotes from languages other than English have been translated by Ingebjørg Midsem Dahl, unless otherwise stated.

Action for ME (2008) *ME 2008: What Progress?* Pamphlet published on the association's website. Found 9th of September 2013, from www.ssb4mesupport.weebly.com/uploads/8/0/5/0/8050248/action_for_me_survey_2008.pdf

Bassett, Jodi. (2009) *Treating ME – Avoiding overexertion.* The Hummingbirds' Foundation for M.E. Downloaded from the Internet 15th of April 2012: www.hfme.org/treatingme.htm

Bassett, Jodi. (2011), *Caring for the ME Patient.* Available from www.lulu.com and www.amazon.com. ISBN: 978-1-4452-9639-5.

Bell, D.S. (1991). *The Disease of a Thousand Names.* Massachusetts: Perseus Books. ISBN: 9992291141.

Bell, D.S., Robinson, M.Z., Pollard, J., Robinson, T., & Floyd, B. (1999). *A Parents' Guide to CFIDS. How To Be An Advocate For Your Child With Chronic Fatigue Immune Dysfunction Syndrome.* Binghampton, NY: The Haworth Medical Press. ISBN: 0789007118.

Bell, D.S. (2001). *Thirteen-Year Follow-Up of Children and Adolescents with Chronic Fatigue Syndrome.* Pediatrics, Vol. 107, nr. 5, 1. May.

Bell, D.S. (2011). *25-Year Follow-Up in Chronic Fatigue Syndrome: Rising Incapacity.* Talk by Dr. Bell for The Massachusetts CFIDS/ME & FM Associations, summarised by Joan Livingston. Retrieved 29 August 2013, from www.masscfids.org/resource-library/3/311

Berge, T., Dehli, L & Fjerstad, E. (2014). *Energityvene – Utmattelse i sykdom og hverdag.* Oslo: H. Aschehoug & Co. (W. Nygaard).

Berne, K. Ph.D. (1995) *CFS and Self-Esteem.* Tape. 2207 E. Ivy Mesa in Arizona 85213.

Berne, K. Ph.D. (1995). *Running on Empty: A complete guide to chronic fatigue syndrome (CFIDS).* New York, NY: Hunter House Publishers.

Bjørkum, T., Wang, C.E.A., & Waterloo, K. (2009). *Pasienterfaringer med ulike tiltak ved kronisk utmattelsessyndrom.* Tidsskrift for Den norske legeforening, 2009 (12).

Black, C.D. & McCully, K.K. (2005). *Time Course of Exercise Induced Alterations in Daily Activity in Chronic Fatigue Syndrome.* Dynamic Medicine, 4 (10). Downloaded from the Internet 23.06.10: www.dynamic-med.com/content/pdf/1476-5918-4-10.pdf

Borg, V. (1986). *Avspenning Autogen Trening.* NCB, AB Records A/S.

Bringsli, G., Gilje, A., Getz Wold, B.K. (2013). *ME-syke I Norge – Fortsatt bortgjemt?* Norges ME forening (The Norwegian ME Association) Retrieved 18.03.2018, from http://me-forskning.no/wp-content/uploads/2013/06/ME-foreningensBrukerunders%C3%B8kelse.pdf

Brotherston, N.E. (2001). *Adolescence and Myalgic Encephalomyelitis/Chronic Fatigue Syndrome: Journeys with the Dragon.* New York, NY: The Haworth Medical Press. ISBN: 9780789008749

Brown, M., Khorana, N. & Jason, L.A. (2010). *The Role of Changes in Activity as a Function of Perceived Available and Expended Energy in Non-Pharmacological Treatment Outcomes for ME/CFS.* Journal of Clinical Psychology, 67(3), 253-260. Downloaded from the Internet 15.10.13 www.ncbi.nlm.nih.gov/pubmed/21254053

Burch, V. & Penman, D. (2013). *Mindfulness for Health. A Practical Guide to Relieving Pain, Reducing Stress and Restoring Wellbeing.* Great Britain: Piatkus.

Campbell, B. (2006). *Managing Chronic Fatigue Syndrome and Fibromyalgia.* CSH Press.

Campbell, B. (2010). *Managing Chronic Fatigue Syndrome and Fibromyalgia.* CSH Press. Can be read free of charge on this website. Downloaded 07.10.2013 www.cfidsselfhelp.org/library/managing-chronic-fatigue-syndrome-and-fibromyalgia

Campling, F., Sharpe, M. (2008). *Chronic Fatigue Syndrome – The Facts.* Oxford University Press.

Carruthers, B.M., Jain, A.K., De Meirleir, K.L., Peterson, D.L., Klimas, N.G., Lerner, A.M., Bested, A.C., Flor-Henry, P., Joshi, P., Powles, A.C.P., Sherkey, J.A., & van de Sande, M.I. (2003). *Myalgic Encephalomyelitis/Chronic Fatigue Syndrome: Clinical Working Case Definition, Diagnostic and Treatment Protocols.* Journal of Chronic Fatigue Syndrome, 11 (1), 7-115. Downloaded from the Internet 23.06.10: www. phoenixrising.me/wp-content/uploads/Canadian-definition.pdf

Carruthers, B.et al. (2011). *Myalgic Encephalomyelitis: International Consensus Criteria.* Journal of Internal Medicine, 20 July 2011.

Carruthers, B.et al. (2011). *Consensus Primer for Medical Practitioners.* Downloaded from the Internet 06.04.2017: www.investinme.org/Documents/Guidelines/Myalgic%20Encephalomyelitis%20International%20Consensus%20Primer%20-2012-11-26.pdf

Chamber, D., Bagnall, A., Hempell, S., Forbes, C. *Interventions for the Treatment, Management and Rehabilitation of Patients with Chronic Fatigue Syndrome/Myalgic Encephalomyelitis: An Updated Systematic Review.* (2006), Journal of the Royal Society of Medicine, vol. 99 nr. 10.

Colby, J. (1996). *ME: The New Plague.* Peterborough (UK): First and Best in Education Ltd. ISBN: 1860832156.

Colby, J. (1999). *Zoë's Win.* Dome Vision, UK. ISBN: 0953733009

Colby, J. (2001). *Ten Points on the Education of Children with ME.* Tymes Magazine 36-2001.

Collinge, W. (1993). *Recovering from Chronic Fatigue Syndrome: A Guide to Self-Empowerment.* New York: The Body Press/Perigee. This book can the read free of charge on the Internet.

Collinge, W. (1995) *Recovering from Chronic Fatigue Syndrome.* Souvenir Press Ltd. ISBN: 039951807X.

Collingridge, E. (2010). *Severe ME/CFS: A Guide to Living.* Milton Keynes, UK: Association of Young People with M.E. (AYME). Can be ordered from Action for M.E. www.actionforme.org.uk or www.severeme.info. Links were correct as of November 8th 2017.

Cox, D. & Findley, L. (1994). *Is Chronic Fatigue Syndrome Treatable in an NHS Environment?* Clinical Rehabilitation – CLIN REHABIL. 01/1994; 8(1):76-80.

Cox, D. & Findley, L. (1998). *The Management of Chronic Fatigue Syndrome in an Inpatient Setting: Presentation of an Approach and Perceived Outcome.* British Journal of Occupational Therapy. 08/1998; 61(9):405-409.

Cox, D. & Findley, L. (2000). *Severe and Very Severe Patients with Chronic Fatigue Syndrome.* Journal of Chronic Fatigue Syndrome 01/1999; 7(3):33-47.

Cox, D. (2000). *Occupational Therapy and Chronic Fatigue Syndrome.* Whurr Publishers. ISBN: 1861561555.

Cox, D. et al. (On behalf of PACE Trial Management Group). (2004). *Manual for Therapists Adaptive Pacing Therapy (APT) for CFS/ME.* Downloaded from the Internet 08.10.2013. www.qmul.ac.uk/wolfson/media/wolfson/current-projects/2.apt-participant-manual.pdf

De Meirleir, K. (2010). Personal communication.

Donoghue, P.J. & Siegel, M.E. (1992). *Sick and Tired of Feeling Sick and Tired: Living with Invisible Chronic Illness.* New York, NY: W.W. Norton & Company, Inc.

Edwards, C.R., Thompson, A.R., Blair, A. (2007). *An 'Overwhelming Illness': Women's Experiences of Learning to Live with Chronic Fatigue Syndrome/Myalgic Encephalomyelitis.* Journal of Health Psychology. 2007; 12; 203.

Festvåg, L., Sparre, M., Opheim, A., & Stanghelle, J.K. (2001). *For utmattet til å trene? Qigong i behandlingen av personer med myalgisk encefalopati/chronic fatigue syndrome.* (Too Exhausted to Exercise? Qigoing in the Treatment of People with Myalgic Encephalomyelitis/Chronic Fatigue Syndrome) Sluttrapport til Helse og rehabilitering. 2001/3/0307. Downloaded 10.11.2017 from www.me-foreningen.info/wp-content/uploads/2016/09/Fysioterapeuten-Qigong-2006.pdf. English summary at the end of the document.

Franklin, A. (1990). *Professional Guides: The Doctor's Guide to ME in Children and Young People.* The Young ME Sufferers Trust. Downloaded from the Internet 23.06.10: www.tymestrust.org/pdfs/drguide.pdf

Friedberg, F. (1995). *Coping with Chronic Fatigue Syndrome: Nine Things You Can Do.* Oakland, CA: New Harbinger Publications.

Friedberg, F. & Jason, L.A. (1998). *Understanding Chronic Fatigue Syndrome: An Empirical Guide to Assessment and Treatment*. Washington, DC: American Psychological Association. ISBN: 9781557985118.

Friedberg, F. (2002). *Does Graded Activity Increase Activity? A Case Study of Chronic Fatigue Syndrome*. J. Behav. Ther. & Exp. Psychiat. 33 (2002) 203–215.

Friedberg, F. et al. (2012).*ME/CFS: A Primer for Clinical Practitioners*. International Association for Chronic Fatigue Syndrome/Myalgic Encephalomyelitis. New York, USA. Downloaded from the Internet 09.10.2013. www.iacfsme.org/portals/0/pdf/primerfinal3.pdf

Gallagher, A.M., Coldrick, A.R., Hedge, B., Weir, W.R.C., White, P.D. (2005). *Is The Chronic Fatigue Syndrome An Exercise Phobia? A Case Control Study*. Journal of Psychological Research 58, 367-373.

Garde, M. (1999). Personal communication.

Gladwell, P.W., Pheby, D., Rodriques, T. & Poland, F. (2013). *Use of an Online Survey to Explore Positive and Negative Outcomes of Rehabilitation for People with CFS/ME*. Disability and rehabilitation. Epub ahead of print. Retrieved 07.09. 2013, from www.ncbi.nlm.nih.gov/pubmed/23735013

Goudsmit, E.M. (1996).*The Psychological Aspects and Management of Chronic Fatigue Syndrome*. Department of Human Sciences, Brunel University. Retrieved 09.10.2013, from bura.brunel.ac.uk/handle/2438/4283

Goudsmit, E.M. & Howes, S. (2008). *Pacing: A Strategy to Improve Energy Management in Chronic Fatigue Syndrome*. Health Psychology Update, 17 (1), 46–52.

Goudsmit, E.M., Ho-Yen, D.O. & Dancey, C.P. (2009). Learning to *Cope with Chronic Illness. Efficacy of a Multi-Component Treatment for People with Chronic Fatigue Syndrome*. Patient Education and Counselling, 77, 231-236.

Goudsmit, E.M. & Howes, S. (2010). *Pacing: An Additional Strategy to Manage Fatigue in Chronic Fatigue Syndrome*. Retrieved 23.06.10, from www.axfordsabode.org.uk/me/pacing.htm

Goudsmit, E.M., Nijs, J., Jason, L.A. & Wallman, K.E. (2012). *Pacing as a Strategy to Improve Energy Management in Myalgic Encephalomyelitis/Chronic Fatigue Syndrome: A Consensus Document*. Disability and Rehabilitation, 34 (13), 1140-1147.

Gow, J.W., Hagan, S., Herzyk, P., Cannon, C., Behan, P.O., & Chaudhuri, A. (2009). *A Gene Signature for Post-Infectious Chronic Fatigue Syndrome*. BMC Medical Genomics, 2 (38). Downloaded from the Internet 23.06.10: www.biomedcentral.com/content/pdf/1755-8794-2-38.pdf

Hareide, L. (2007), *Mening og mestring,* Masteroppgave ved Psykologisk institutt, Universitetet i Oslo

Helsedirektoratet (06/2013). *Nasjonal veileder – Pasienter med CFS/ME: Utredning, diagnostikk, behandling, rehabilitering, pleie og omsorg*. (Norwegian Department of Health, National Guideline – Patients with CFS/ME: Diagnosis, treatment, rehabilitation and care.)

Retrieved 17.03.18 from https://helsedirektoratet.no/Lists/Publikasjoner/Attachments/396/IS-1944-Nasjonal-Veileder-CFS-ME-Hovedversjon.pdf

Hickie, I., Davenport, T.A., Wakefield, D., Vollmer-Conna, U., Cameron, B., Vernon, S.D. et al. (2006). *Post-Infective and Chronic Fatigue Syndromes Precipitated by Viral and Non-Viral Pathogens: Prospective Cohort Study. British Medical Journal, 333 (7568), 575.*

Ho-Yen, D.O. (2003). *Better Recovery from Viral Illnesses.* Inverness: Dodona Books. ISBN: 0951109030.

Ho-Yen, D.O. *How To Float (And Not Drown!)* in *Times Magazine, 2000* nr. 31.

Hvenegaard, V. (1999). Kastanieblomsten: En familie med ME/CFS (Kronisk træthedssyndrom). (The Chestnut Flower: A Family with ME/CFS Chronic Fatigue Syndrome) Nyborg: Hvenegaards Forlag.

Hyde, B.M., Goldstein, J., Levine, P., & (Eds.) (1992). *The Clinical and Scientific Basis of Myalgic Encephalomyelitis/Chronic Fatigue Syndrome.* Ottawa: The Nightingale Research Foundation. ISBN: 0969566204.

Iger, Linda Miller, PhD. *The View from the Other Side of the Couch: Treating Memory and Concentration Losses.* The CEFIDS Chronicle Physicians' Forum. Volume 1, Issue 2, August 1991.

Jason, L.A., Melrose, H., Lerman, A. et.al. (1999) *Managing Chronic Fatigue Syndrome: Overview and Case Study.* Official Journal of the American Association of Occupational Health Nurses, 47(1), 17-21. Retrieved 15.10.2013, from www.ncbi.nlm.nih.gov/pubmed/10205371

Jason, L.A. (2007) *Non-Pharmacologic Interventions for CFS: A Randomized Trial.* Journal of Clinical Psychology in Medical Settings, 14(4), 275-296. Retrieved 15.10.2013, from www.link.springer.com/article/10.1007/s10880-007-9090-7

Jason, L.A., Muldowney, K. & Torres-Harding, S. (2008). *The Energy Envelope Theory and Myalgic Encephalomyelitis/Chronic Fatigue Syndrome.* Official Journal of the American Association of Occupational Health Nurses. 56(5), 189-95. Retrieved 15.10. 2013, from www.ncbi.nlm.nih.gov/pubmed/18578185

Jason, L.A., Benton, M. (2009). *The Impact of Energy Modulation on Physical Functioning and Fatigue Severity among Patients with ME/CFS.* Patient Education and Counselling. 77(2), 237–241. Retrieved 15.10.2013, from www.ncbi.nlm.nih.gov/pmc/articles/PMC2767446

For more studies by Jason, see also Brown et.al. (2010) and Goudsmit et.al. (2012).

Johnston et al. (2014) *A Comparison of Health Status in Patients Meeting Alternative Definitions for Chronic Fatigue Syndrome/Myalgic Encephalomyelitis.* Health and Quality of Life Outcomes 2014, 12:64. www.hqlo.com/content/pdf/1477-7525-12-64.pdf

Jönsson, S. (2005). *Myalgisk encefalopati (ME) - Informasjon til skole.* Norges Myalgisk Encefalopati Forening. Retrieved 17.03.18, from www.udir.no/PageFiles/87248/ME-info-til-skole.pdf

Kindlon, T. (2011). *Reporting of Harms Associated with Graded Exercise Therapy and Cognitive Behavioural Therapy in Myalgic Encephalomyelitis/Chronic Fatigue Syndrome.* Bulletin of the IACFS/ME. 19(2), 59-111.

Kongsberg og Nummedal PPT (Kongsberg and Nummedal Educational Psychology Service, Norway). www.ppt-ot.no/no/utfordringer_og_vansker/medisinske_problemstillinger. juni 2012.

Kreyberg, S. (2007). Erfaringer med pleie i institusjon ved alvorlig myalgisk encefalopati (ME). (Experiences of Institutional Care of Patients with Severe ME). *Norsk Tidsskrift for Sykepleierforskning*, 9:2, 16-26. (With English summary).

Kreyberg, S. (2008). *ME – en sykdom i tiden.* Published through and available from www.lulu.com. ID: 5214629

Kreyberg, S. *12 Basic Rules of Handling ME.* Retrieved 26.11.16 from www.totoneimbehl.wordpress.com/skjemainfo-om-me-g93-3/12-grunnregler-ved-sykdommen-myalgisk-encefalopati-me/12-basic-rules-for-handling-myalgic-encephalopathy-me

Larun, L., Malterud, K. (2007). *Identity and Coping Experiences in Chronic Fatigue Syndrome: A Synthesis of Qualitative Studies.* Elsevier. DOI: 10.1016/j.pec.2007.06.008

Macintyre, A. (1998). *ME – Post Viral Fatigue Syndrome - How To Live With It.* London: Thorsons Health. ISBN: 0722526245

Maes, M., Twisk, F.N. (2009). *Chronic Fatigue Syndrome: La Bête Noire of the Belgian Health Care System.* Neuroendocrinology Letters, 30(3), 300–311. Retrieved 15.10.2013, from www.ncbi.nlm.nih.gov/pubmed/19855351

Maes, M., Twisk, F.N. (2010). *Chronic Fatigue Syndrome: Harvey and Wessely's (Bio)Psychosocial Model Versus a Bio(Psychosocial) Model Based on Inflammatory and Oxidative and Nitrosative Stress Pathways.* BMC Medicine, 8 (35). Retrieved 23.06.10, from www.biomedcentral.com/content/pdf/1741-7015-8-35.pdf

The ME Association UK. (2008). Summary of membership survey. *ME Essential (Spring 2008)*, 8.

The ME Association (2010) *Managing my ME. What People with ME/CFS and their Carers Want from the UK's Health and Social Services. The Results of the ME Association's Major Survey of Illness Management Requirements.* The ME Association. Supplement to ME essential, Issue No 114.

Moss, J.I. (1995). *Somebody Help ME - A Self-Help Guide for Young Sufferers from Myalgic Encephalomyelitis and Their Families.* Milton Keynes, UK: Sunbow Books. ISBN: 0952578301.

Moss, J.I. (2008). *A Ray of Hope.* Sunbow Books. ISBN: 0952578336.

Myhill, S., Booth, N.E., & McLaren-Howard, J. (2009). *Chronic Fatigue Syndrome and Mitochondrial Dysfunction.* International Journal of Clinical and Experimental Medicine, 2 (1), 1–16. Retrieved 23.06.10, from www.ijcem.com/files/IJCEM812001.pdf

Nijs, J., Vanherberghen, K., Duquet, W., De Meirleir, K. (2004). *Chronic Fatigue Syndrome: Lack of Association between Pain-Related Fear of Movement and Exercise Capacity and Disability.* Phys Ther. 2004 Aug; 84(8):696-705.

Owen, Lois G. (2010). *Bed without Boundaries: Therapeutic Activities for Chronically Ill People.* UK: Arts in Action Publications.

Pemberton, S., Berry, C. (2009). *Fighting Fatigue: Managing the Symptoms of CFS/ME.* Hammersmith Press Limited. ISBN: 1905140282.

Pheby, D. & Saffron, L. (2009). *Risk factors for Severe ME/CFS.* Biology and Medicine, 1 (4), 50–74

Pheby, D. (2011). *GET, GAT and Exercise on Prescription Survey Results.* InterAction, 75, 11-13

Pierce, S. & Pierce, P.W. (2009). *The Physiology of Exercise Intolerance in Patients with Myalgic Encephalomyelitis (ME) and the Utility of Graded Exercise Therapy.* Journal of Invest in ME, 2 (2), 55–60. 18–22.

Pinxsterhuis, I. (2008). *Myalgisk Encefalopati og utførelse av daglige aktviteter. Om å leve med "dårlige" batterier.* (ME and Performance of Daily Activities. Living with 'Poor' Batteries.) Master i helsefagvitenskap. (Master's degree thesis) Seksjon for helsefag. Det medisinske fakultetet, Universitetet i Oslo. Autum 2008. (With English summary.) Retrieved 16.10.2013 from https://www.duo.uio.no/handle/10852/28543

Pinxsterhuis, I. (2010). *Aktivitetsavpassing og energiøkonomisering/energibesparende metoder.* Retrieved 18.08.2013 from https://oslo-universitetssykehus.no/seksjon-avdeling/PublishingImages/avdelinger/medisinsk-klinikk/geriatrisk-avdeling/cfsme-senteret/Aktivitetsavpasning%20og%20energi%C3%B8konomisering%20energibesparende%20metoder%202017.pdf

Pinxsterhuis, I. (2011). *Hvilke faktorer kan føre til forbedring av aktivitetsnivå hos de aller sykeste?* Foredrag ved CFS/ME Erfaringskonferanse for helsepersonell. Helse Sør-Øst 11. november 2011. Referert av Cathrine Eide Westerby. Retrieved 17.03.2018, from http://www.serendipitycat.no/wp-content/uploads/2011/11/Referat-Erfaringskonferanse-CFSME-Helse-S%C3%B8r-%C3%98st-111111-_Fullversjon_.pdf

Price, J.R. & Couper, J. (1998). *Cognitive Behavior Therapy for Chronic Fatigue Syndrome in Adults (Review).* The Cochrane Collaboration. Retrieved 02.08.2014, from www.thecochranelibrary.com

Ramsay, A.M. (1988). *Myalgic Encephalomyelitis and Post-viral Fatigue States: The Saga of Royal Free Disease.* London: Gower Medical Publishing. ISBN: 0906923999

Ramsay, A.M. (1986). *A Baffling Syndrome with a Tragic Aftermath.* Retrieved 17.11.2017 from www.cfstreatmentguide.com/blog/myalgic-encephalomyelitis-a-baffling-syndrome-with-a-tragic-aftermath-by-a-melvin-ramsay

Richardson, J. (2001). *Enteroviral and Toxin Mediated Myalgic Encephalomyelitis/Chronic Fatigue Syndrome and other Organ Pathologies.* New York: The Haworth Press. ISBN: 0-7890-1128-X

Shepherd, C. (1999). *Living with ME, the Chronic/Post-Viral Fatigue Syndrome*. London: Vermillion, Ebury Press. ISBN-10: 009181679

Shepherd, C. (1998). *Living with ME, the Chronic/Post-Viral Fatigue Syndrome ME*. London: Vermillion, Ebury Press. Kapittel 8: *The Glass Ceiling*. Times Magazine (nr. 43, vår 2003).

Shropshire Enablement Team (2009). *Setting the Pace*. Shropshire Enablement Team. ISBN: 9780956170606

Snell, C.R. (2013). *Discriminative Validity of Metabolic and Workload Measurements to Identify Individuals with Chronic Fatigue Syndrome*. American Physical Therapy Association, 2013. Retrieved 03.01.2014, from www.ncbi.nlm.nih.gov/pubmed/23813081

Sparre, M. (2007). *Å møte mennesker med ME – veiledning og behandling*. Foredrag på fagdag i regi av Sølvskottberget rehabiliteringssenter, Fåberg 31.01.2007. Retrieved 02.04.12 from www.tropos.no

Sparre, M. (2009). *Balansenøkler – om å balansere kroppen og livet*. ISBN: 978-82-991850-1

Twisk, F.N.M. & Maes, M. (2009). *A Review on Cognitive Behavorial Therapy (CBT) and Graded Exercise Therapy (GET) in Myalgic Encephalomyelitis (ME)/Chronic Fatigue Syndrome (CFS): CBT/GET is not only ineffective and not evidence-based, but also potentially harmful for many patients with ME/CFS*. Neuroendocrinology Letters, 39 (3), 284–299.

Twisk, F.N.M. (2014). *The Status of and Future Research into Myalgic Encephalomyelitis and Chronic Fatigue Syndrome: The Need of Accurate Diagnosis, Objective Assessment, and Acknowledging Biological and Clinical Subgroups*. Frontier in Physiology 5: 109. Retrieved 07.03.2014 from www.ncbi.nlm.nih.gov/pubmed/24734022

Vercoulen, J.H.M.M. et al. (1998). *The Persistence of Fatigue in Chronic Fatigue Syndrome and Multiple Sclerosis: Development of a Model*. Journal of Psychosomatic Research, 45, 507-517.

Verrillo, E.F. & Gellman, L.M. (1997). *Chronic Fatigue Syndrome: A Treatment Guide*. New York: St. Martin's Griffin. ISBN: 1-57626-053-4

Verrillo, E.F. (2012) *Chronic fatigue Syndrome: A treatment guide*. Self-published. ASIN: B009B9X36Y Available from: www.amazon.com/gp/product/B009B9X36Y/ref=kinw_myk_ro_title

Wade, C. (2004). *Surviving Severe ME*. Association of Young People with ME (AYME). Downloaded from the Internet 23.06.10: www.survivingsevereme.com

White, P. et.al (2011). *Comparison of Adaptive Pacing Therapy, Cognitive Behaviour Therapy, Graded Exercise Therapy, and Specialist Medical Care for Chronic Fatigue Syndrome (PACE): A Randomised Trial*. The Lancet, 377(9768), 823-836. Retrieved 03.10.2013 from www.sciencedirect.com/science/article/pii/S0140673611600962

Williams, Z. (2002). *The ME Tips Collection*. Irish ME/CFS Support Group. Downloaded from Internet 23.06.10. www.trevwilliams.co.uk/metips/home.html. Also available from: www.metips.co.uk.

SOURCES OF PATIENT QUOTES

This list contains quotes taken from patient articles and letters found in ME magazines. All patient quotes which do not appear on this list are from personal correspondence. Not all the patient organisations mentioned on the list still exist.

- Abigail Owen (2002). Interaction Issue 41, July 2002. *An ME Clinic Turned my Life Around*, pp 6-8.

- Anna (2002). *I Can't Tell How I Feel*. Cheers, Association of Young People with ME newsletter, nr. 40, Mar/Apr 2002, 35.

- Bryony P. (2007). Letter to the editor. Cheers, Association of Young People with ME newsletter, nr. 72.

- Diane Shortland (2005). *Laughter therapy: Unmissable Events: Shorty's guide to ME Friendly Weddings*. AYME Graduates Newsletter nr. 13, August 2005, (newsletter of a subgroup of Association of Young People with M.E, age 26+), UK, 12–13.

- Isla, Poster from The Young ME Sufferers' Trust, (May 2014). http://tymestrust.org/pdfs/tt25years.pdf

- Joan T. (1999). *ME and Joan's Story*. Cheers, Association of Young People with ME newsletter, nr. 24, July/August 1999, 24.

- Kathryn D. (2000). *Rest and Relaxation for Recovery*. Cheers, Association of Young People with ME newsletter, nr. 32, December 2000, 27.

- Shula F. (2006). *My Experience of Being Me with ME*. AYME Graduates Newsletter, May 2006 (newsletter of a subgroup of Association of Young People with M.E, age 26+), UK, 2–3.

- Veness, B. *How I Use Pacing to Manage CFS*. Retrieved 18.08.2013, from www.cfidsselfhelp.org/library/how-i-use-pacing-manage-cfs

If you wish to find out more about ME than what you can find on this reference list, you can find summaries of 2,000 articles on ME Research's UK website: www.meresearch.org.uk/information/research-database.

A series of considerably shorter summaries of ME research from 1955 until the present, from a spectrum of medical subspecialties, can be found in Professor Malcom Hooper's document *Magical Medicine, How to Make a Disease Disappear,* which can be found at:

www.investinme.org/Article400%20Magical%20Medicine.htm. The research summaries start on page 98. The links were correct as per 26.10.17.

WORKSHEETS 1-10

All of these worksheets can be printed out from the author's website at www.pacinginfo.eu.

Worksheet 1 – Experimentation Sheet

Worksheet 2 – Activity Scale for Simple Activity Diary

Worksheet 3 – Simple Activity Diary

Worksheet 4 – Detailed Activity Diary

Worksheet 5 – Graph Sheet for Simple Activity Diary

Worksheet 6 – Analysis Sheet

Worksheet 7 – Priority Sheet

Worksheet 8 – How to Make a Graph from a Detailed Activity Diary

Worksheet 9 – Graph Sheet for Detailed Activity Diary

Worksheet 10 – Example of an Invitation to a Virtual Party

WORKSHEET 1 – EXPERIMENTATION SHEET

ACTIVITY	NONE	NONE	NONE	SLIGHT	MODERATE	SEVERE	VERY SEVERE	RELAPSE
	Degree of symptom increase (fill in number of minutes)							
Socialising with one person								
Socialising with several people								
Telephone call								
Watching TV								
Showering								
Washing the dishes								
Driving								
Shopping								
Walking								
Reading								
Listening to music								
Brushing teeth								
Dressing								
Cooking								
Meals								
Craft activities								
Handwriting								
Typing								
Internet								
Cleaning								
Tidying								
Texting								
Caring for/being with children								
Work/school								
Public transportation								
Exercising								
Playing indoors								
Playing outdoors								
Sitting								
Standing								

ACTIVITY	NONE	NONE	NONE	SLIGHT	MODERATE	SEVERE	VERY SEVERE	RELAPSE
	Degree of symptom increase (fill in number of minutes)							
Fill in your own activities below								

WORKSHEET 2 – ACTIVITY SCALE FOR SIMPLE ACTIVITY DIARY

Compare today's activity level with the descriptions below. Write the most suitable number in your diary. If you fall between two levels, for instance 40 and 50, you can write the number in between in your diary, 45. Rate today's symptom level on a scale from 0 to 10, where 0 signifies no symptoms, and 10 signifies very severe symptoms. Write this number as well in the diary.

HEALTHY	100 Work or study full time without difficulty, plus enjoy a normal social life and exercise normally. Back to climbing mountains on weekends.
VERY MILD	95 Can manage work or school full time. Social life and a bit of exercise, but have to be careful with physical activity. Somewhat poorer stamina than healthy people.
MILD	90 Considerably better stamina compared to 80%. Can work or study full time, but with some difficulty. Can go out at night without paying dearly for it afterwards, but is still more tired than normal the next day. 80 Can get through the day without problems, so long as one gets sufficient sleep and does not do too much. Full-time work or study is difficult, especially if it is a noisy, crowded or busy environment. Can manage part-time work without difficulty, but need more sleep than before.

MODERATE	**70** Can get through the day without a rest break, but need more sleep than healthy people. Daily activity limited. Part-time studying is tiring and may restrict social life. A few hours of part-time work may be possible or working a bit from home. Can manage most household chores and errands with rest afterwards. Have to go to bed early. Can drive short distances. Gentle walking and swimming may be possible. **60** Some days a rest break or nap may be necessary. Can get through the day with short rest periods. Daily activity very limited. Can manage most housework yourself, but this limits other activities. Can drive short distances. Studying with others or work outside the home is very difficult unless one can get different types of support, such as a wheelchair and a room for rest breaks. One to two hours of studying or work in the home may be possible on good days. Quiet, restful social life is possible.
MODERATE TO SEVERE	**50** Need long rest breaks or need to nap. Short, simple (1 hour) home study possible if alternated with quiet, non-active social life. Limited concentration span. Not confined to the house, but unable to walk far without support (100-200 metres). Can manage a short wheelchair ride, short shopping trips or visit a friend. Could manage most household tasks with pacing and breaks, but this would mean sacrificing other activities such as education. **40** Can be up for 2-3 hours at a stretch, but needs as much rest as activity. Can prepare simple meals and do a little light housework. Not confined to the house, but is rarely able to walk more than 50-100 metres, usually with crutches, stick or rollator. Can manage a short wheelchair ride to the shops on a quiet day. Can drive short distances but prefer others to do the driving. Needs 3-4 regular rest breaks during the day. Can only manage one 'large' activity per day, e.g. friend dropping by or short doctor's visit or half an hour home tuition. Require a resting period of one or more days before the next 'large' activity.

SEVERE	**30** Often has a window of 2-3 hours when one can do a bit more, but still needs to rest during this time. Can be up for a while, but cannot move around much. Usually too ill to leave the house, but may be able to manage a short wheelchair ride or a very short walk in the fresh air occasionally. Most of the day resting. Very small activities can be carried out, but homework and home tuition are difficult. Home tuition may be impossible for children at this level. Can do a little light house work, but still needs assistance for many things. **20** May be able to get up for an hour or so, but cannot move around much. Usually unable to leave the house. Confined to bed/sofa most of the day, but able to sit up for a few short periods. Unable to concentrate for more than one hour a day in total, but may be able to read for 5-10 minutes at a time. Needs assistance for all housework.
VERY SEVERE	**10** In bed all day. Can only be up for a maximum of 10 minutes. No travel outside the home. Concentration very difficult. May be able to manage a visitor for 10 minutes at a time. May occasionally be able to be transported lying down to a test that cannot be done at home, but it takes a long time to get over this afterwards. **5** May be able to sit up in bed for very short periods if well supported. Small personal care possible, e.g. it may be possible to wash part of body if washing things are brought to the bed. No TV possible at this stage, but some may be able to cope with a few minutes of quiet music or audio books. A friend can be seen for a minute or so for a hug and a few words. **0** In bed constantly and feels extremely ill even with permanent rest. Almost impossible to be propped up in bed for more than a few minutes. Curtains must be closed and ear plugs are necessary. Unable to care for yourself. Washing has to be done a tiny bit at a time. Eating is extremely difficult. Liquid feed preferred at this stage, little and often. Sometimes nasal feeding tubes are necessary when energy to chew is completely spent. Other people moving around the room is straining. Visitors almost impossible. Speaking is often impossible even to the carer or family. This may be misunderstood as being selectively mute.

This functional ability guide is only meant as a guide. There will always be individual differences. The activities mentioned at each level are only examples.

The scale is a combination and adaptation of two scales, 'Association of Young People with ME's Functional Ability Scale' and the scale in the first edition of *Chronic Fatigue Syndrome – A Treatment Guide* by Lauren M. Gellman and Erica F. Verillo. In the original version both describe ability level and symptom level in one, and both scales assume that people with a high ability level have a low symptom level and vice versa. This means that the scales do not cover all possible variations. For instance, it is possible to do a lot in one day and feel very ill whilst doing it, or do very little and feel relatively okay. To register these nuances one has to assess ability level and symptom level in two separate scales. That is why Chapter 14 recommends that one assesses the symptom level from 0 to 10, but uses the above scale when assessing the activity level. For this reason, I have removed the symptom level in this version of the scale.

WORKSHEET 3 — SIMPLE ACTIVITY DIARY

WEEK:	MONTH:	YEAR:
MONDAY	ACTIVITY LEVEL (0–100):	SYMPTOM LEVEL (0–10):
COMMENTS:		
TUESDAY	ACTIVITY LEVEL (0–100):	SYMPTOM LEVEL (0–10):
COMMENTS:		
WEDNESDAY	ACTIVITY LEVEL (0–100):	SYMPTOM LEVEL (0–10):
COMMENTS:		
THURSDAY	ACTIVITY LEVEL (0–100):	SYMPTOM LEVEL (0–10):
COMMENTS:		
FRIDAY	ACTIVITY LEVEL (0–100):	SYMPTOM LEVEL (0–10):
COMMENTS:		
SATURDAY	ACTIVITY LEVEL (0–100):	SYMPTOM LEVEL (0–10):
COMMENTS:		
SUNDAY	ACTIVITY LEVEL (0–100):	SYMPTOM LEVEL (0–10):
COMMENTS:		

WORKSHEET 4 — DETAILED ACTIVITY DIARY

SYMPTOM LEVEL BEFORE ACTIVITY (0-10):	TYPE OF ACTIVITY OR REST:	TIME:	SYMPTOMS:	SYMPTOM LEVEL AFTER ACTIVITY (0-10):	GRADE (0–4) (SEE CHAPTER 16)	POINTS (SEE CHAPTER 16)

Continued on reverse

OBSERVATIONS			NOTES
Sleep (hours):		*Other observations:*	
Meals (number):			
Menstruation (x):			
Weather: S(un), O(vercast), R(ain), T(hunder):			
Noise/sounds (0-10):			
Food changes (note below):			
SYMPTOMS (0-10)		*Other symptoms:*	
Fatigue/exhaustion:			
Malaise:			
Sleep disturbance:			
Muscle twitching:			
Numbness and tingling:			
Allergy (what, write notes below):			
Concentration problems:			
Memory problems:			
Oversensitivity:			
Light:			
Noise:			
Touch:			
Smells:			
Pulse/blood pressure/shortness of breath:			
Dizziness:			
Sore throat:			
Nausea:			
Diarrhoea/constipation:			
Thirst/hunger:			
Pain/discomfort (where):			

WORKSHEET 5 – GRAPH SHEET FOR SIMPLE ACTIVITY DIARY

Month:_____ Year:____

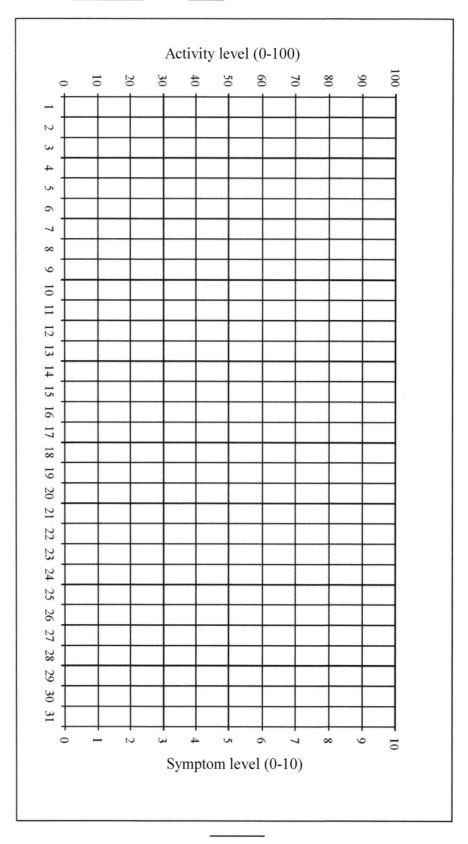

WORKSHEET 6 — ANALYSIS SHEET

+ WORSENING OF SYMPTOMS	0 NO CHANGE IN SYMPTOMS	— IMPROVEMENT OF SYMPTOMS

Source: Vidyamala Burch and Danny Penman, *Mindfulness for Health* (2013).

WORKSHEET 7 — PRIORITY SHEET

JOBS I *HAVE* TO DO:	JOBS I ENJOY:
JOBS OTHERS CAN DO:	**JOBS I DO NOT HAVE TO DO:**

WORKSHEET 8 — HOW TO MAKE A GRAPH FROM A DETAILED ACTIVITY DIARY

In the following, a method for making a graph from a detailed activity diary is described. The method is a combination of two different techniques. The groups of activities shown in Figure 1 are taken from the American ME specialist Dr. David Bell's checklist for school nurses. The method for transforming the activity diary into numbers comes from the book *Somebody Help ME* by Jill Moss.

FIGURE 1: DOCTOR BELL'S RATING SCALE FOR ACTIVITIES

TYPE OF ACTIVITY	GRADE	EXAMPLES OF ACTIVITY
Sleep	0	
Rest	0	Relaxation also counts as rest, except for very ill patients.
Light activity	1	Light reading, watching TV, etc.
Moderate activity indoors	2	Homework, home tuition, meals, dishwashing, etc.
Moderate activity outdoors	3	School, walking, shopping, etc.
Strenuous activities	4	Sport, exercise, cleaning, etc.

In order to turn the activities into numbers to plot on the graph, you find out which of the groups in the table the activity belongs to. You then multiply the length of the activity in minutes by the grade of the activity.

For instance, an hour of watching TV while lying on the sofa will be 60 minutes x 1 = 60 points, while a half hour shopping trip will be 30 minutes x 3 = 90 points. You then add up all the numbers to get a total sum for the day. Do not despair if you have difficulties with the calculations. Use a calculator or ask somebody to help you if necessary. An example of how to calculate the total sum for the day is shown in Figure 2.

FIGURE 2: EXAMPLE OF POINT CALCULATION

Washing and dressing	15 minutes	x 2	= 30 points
Breakfast	15 minutes	x 2	= 30 points
Rest	1 hour		
Read newspaper in bed	15 minutes	x 1	= 15 points
Rest	1 hour		
Lunch	20 minutes	x 2	= 40 points
Rest	1 hour		
Walk	5 minutes	x 3	= 15 points
Rest	1 hour		
Craft activity	10 minutes	x 2	= 20 points
Rest	1 hour		
Dinner	30 minutes	x 2	= 60 points
Rest	1 hour		
Watching TV	30 minutes	x 1	= 30 points
Rest	1 hour		
Snack	15 minutes	x 2	= 30 points
Teeth brushing and undressing	10 minutes	x 2	= 20 points
Total sum for the day			= 290 points

This example was deliberately made very simple. Most people probably have a higher activity level. A total sum like the one in Figure 2 does not say anything about whether the activities were spread out sensibly throughout the day. The sum only says something about the total energy expenditure that day. The energy expenditure is also shown in a relatively imprecise way. Bell's way of splitting activities into six groups is a very rough measure, and there will be differences in how exerting one finds the activities within the same group. A precise grouping does not exist, and if it had existed, it would probably have been too complicated to be of practical use. It does not, however, matter all that much that the total sum is not precise. The small differences become apparent when one analyses the diary on a micro and middle level. What we need on the macro level is to see the difference between an evening on the sofa and an evening at a family party. Large differences are clearly visible in Bell's scale.

When one has kept a diary for a few days, one can draw a graph. One can use Worksheet 9: Graph Sheet for Detailed Activity Diary. It is also possible to draw a graph on regular squared paper or on squared paper which fits in the time manager you use. The graph itself is made by marking one point for the activity level and another point for the symptom level each day. When you have marked the points for the next day, you can draw a line between the points for symptom level and a separate one between the points for activity level. After a while you get two lines and can see that there is a connection between the activity level and the symptom level. An example of such a connection is that the symptom level goes up if one does more than one normally does. The purpose of the graph is to see how the activity level develops from day to day and week to week. How to interpret the graph is described in Chapter 16.

WORKSHEET 9 –

GRAPH SHEET FOR DETAILED ACTIVITY DIARY

Month:_____ Year:____

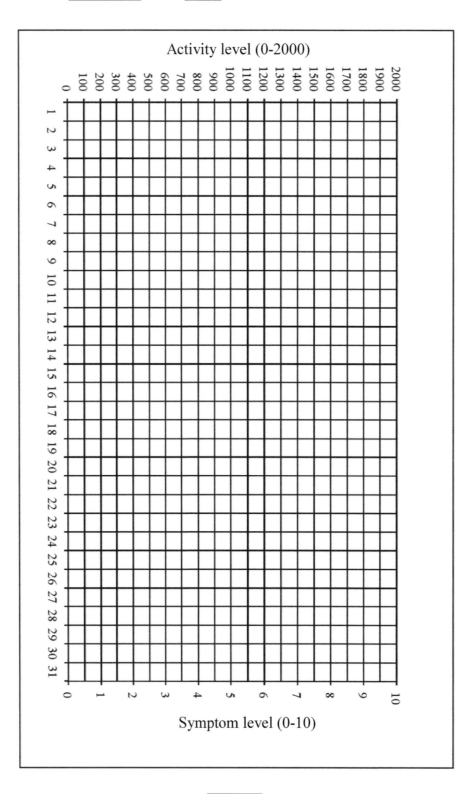

WORKSHEET 10 – EXAMPLE OF AN INVITATION TO A VIRTUAL PARTY

VIRTUAL CHRISTMAS PARTY

You are invited to a virtual Christmas party. Are you unable to go to a normal Christmas party? Do not despair; there will be a Christmas party for us here at Facebook too. Log on in the afternoon or the evening and say hello to the others. This can be done in just as small or large portions as you can cope with. You can also add food and other activities – see below.

Time: (When it suits you)

Place: In your home

Posture: Relaxed (lying flat if you like)

FOOD:

Whatever you can tolerate, but feel free to choose something that puts you in Christmas mood, for instance Christmas tea. If you cannot tolerate Christmas food, go for the cocktail party version: sparkling water and olives.

DRESS CODE:

Santa hats are allowed. Upload a photo of yourself if you decide to dress up as a Christmas tree, reindeer or sleigh.

Decorations are optional, but you can create Christmas ambience with Christmas decorations and Christmas music.

ACTIVITIES:

If you absolutely have to do more than look at the Facebook page and eat something good, you can make Christmas cards, decorations or the like.

LOOKING FORWARD TO SEEING YOU, AND MERRY CHRISTMAS!

PRINTED AND BOUND BY:

Copytech (UK) Limited trading as Printondemand-worldwide,
9 Culley Court, Bakewell Road, Orton Southgate.
Peterborough, PE2 6XD, United Kingdom.
